DONOVAN & WINSLOW
IN
DON'T BE A BULLY

BY MR. A. WITH ANGELA

© 2011 MR. A WITH ANGELA. ALL RIGHTS RESERVED.

NO PART OF THIS BOOK MAY BE REPRODUCED, STORED IN A RETRIEVAL SYSTEM, OR TRANSMITTED BY ANY MEANS WITHOUT THE WRITTEN PERMISSION OF THE AUTHOR.

ISBN 978-0-692-29349-2

LIBRARY OF CONGRESS CONTROL NUMBER: 2011911496
PRINTED IN THE UNITED STATES OF AMERICA

BECAUSE OF THE DYNAMIC NATURE OF THE INTERNET, ANY WEB ADDRESSES OR LINKS CONTAINED IN THIS BOOK MAY HAVE CHANGED SINCE PUBLICATION AND MAY NO LONGER BE VALID. THE VIEWS EXPRESSED IN THIS WORK ARE SOLELY THOSE OF THE AUTHOR AND DO NOT NECESSARILY REFLECT THE VIEWS OF THE PUBLISHER, AND THE PUBLISHER HEREBY DISCLAIMS ANY RESPONSIBILITY FOR THEM.

DEDICATED TO ABUSED CHILDREN
EVERYWHERE

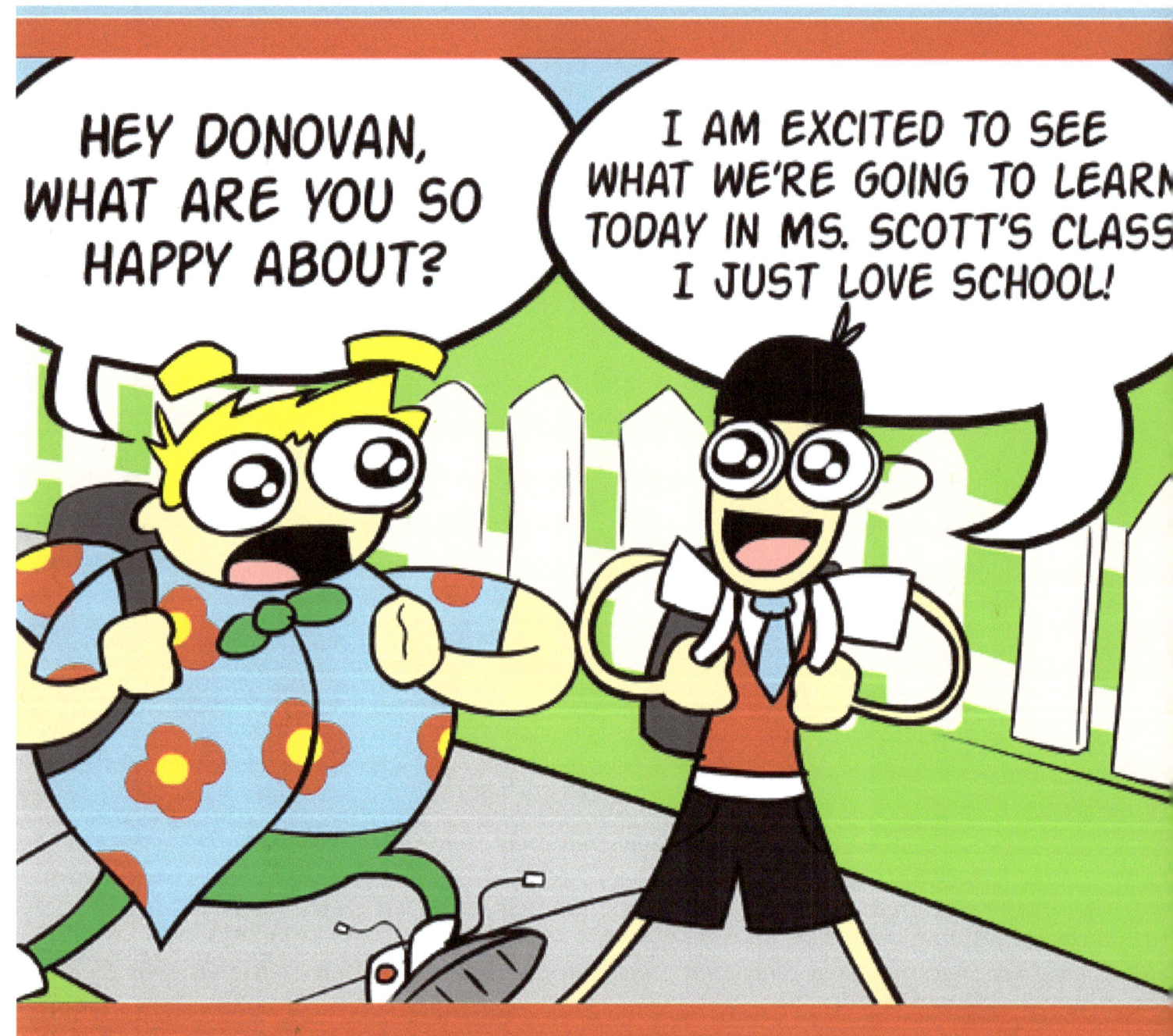

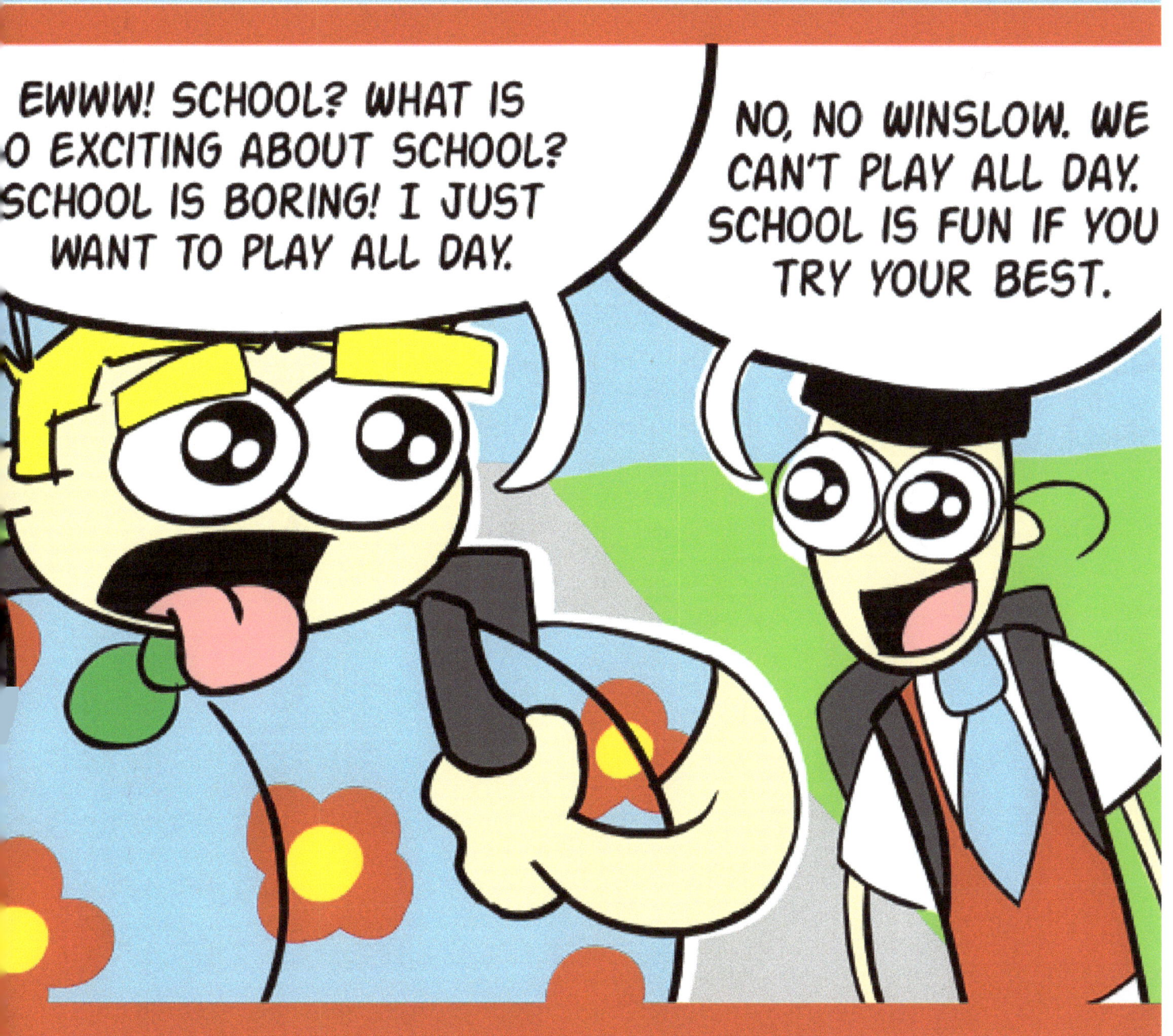

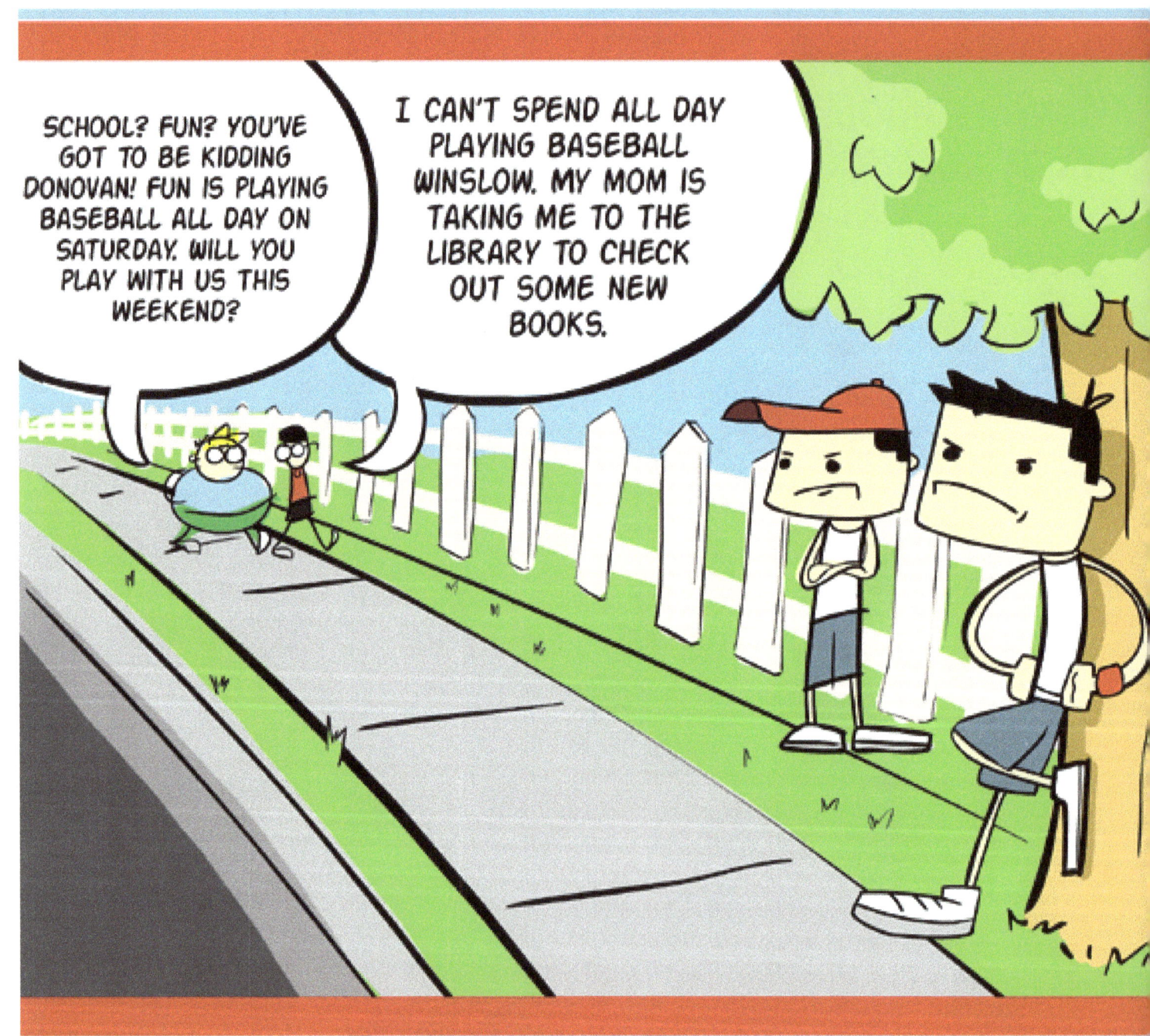

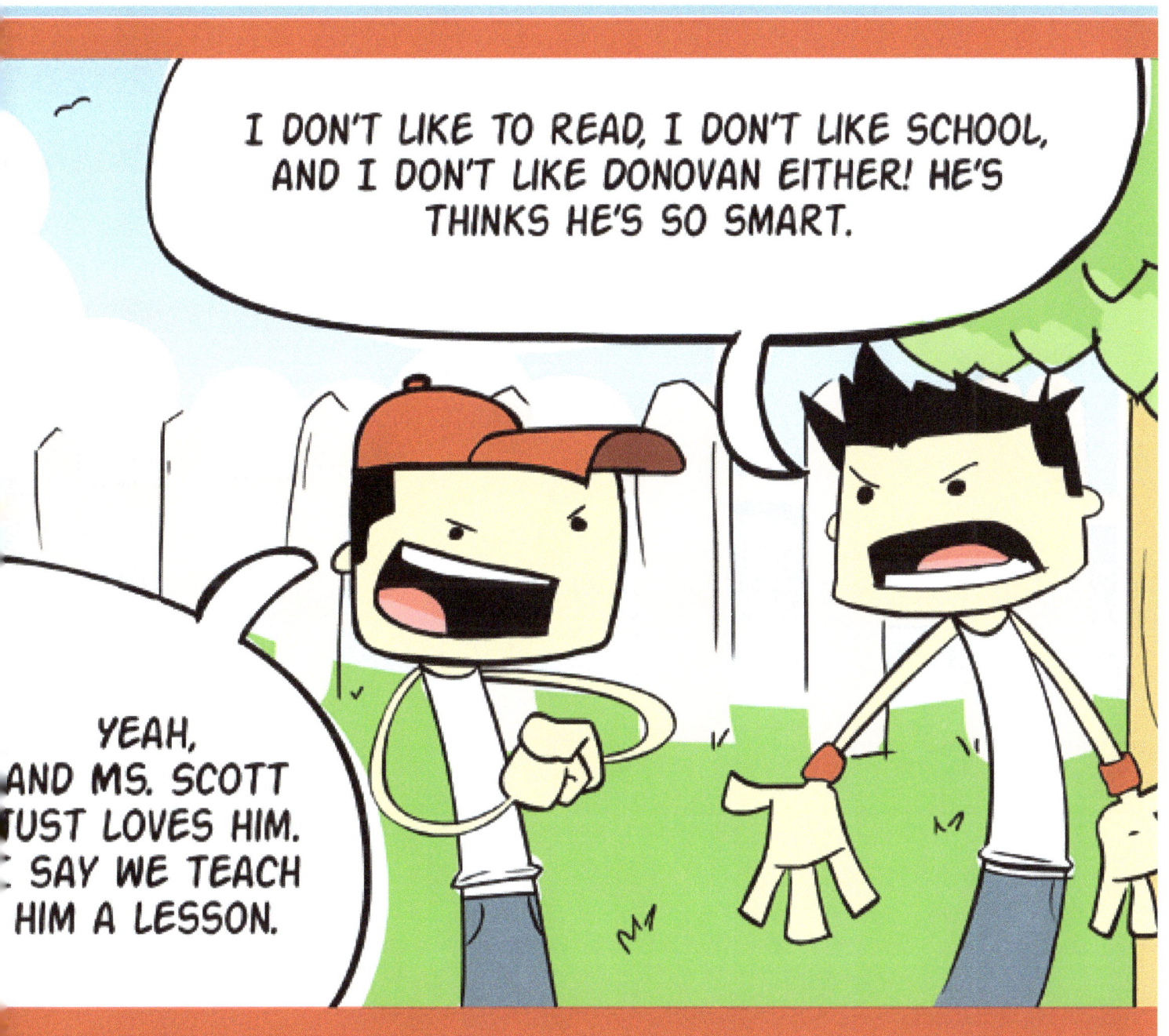

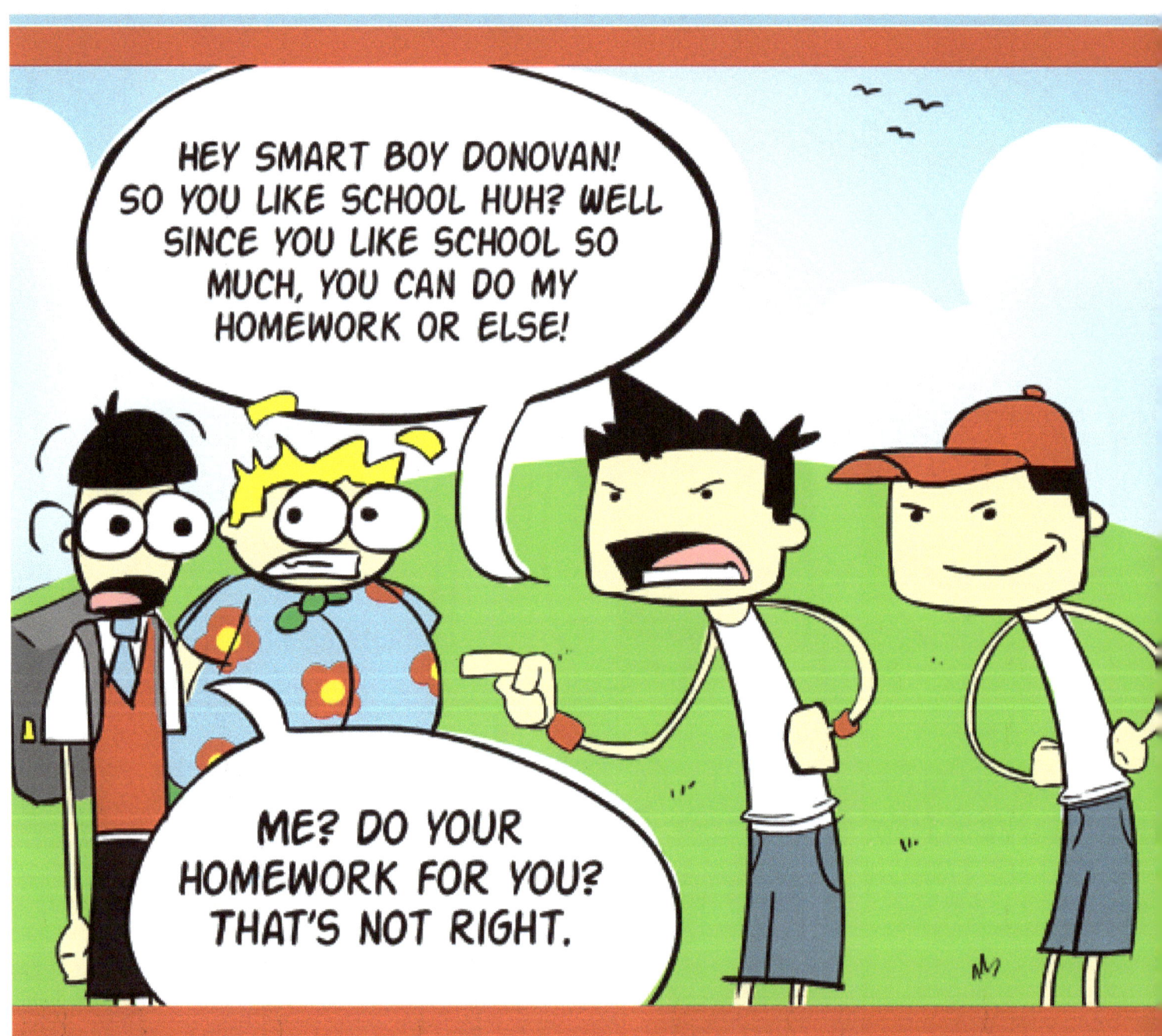

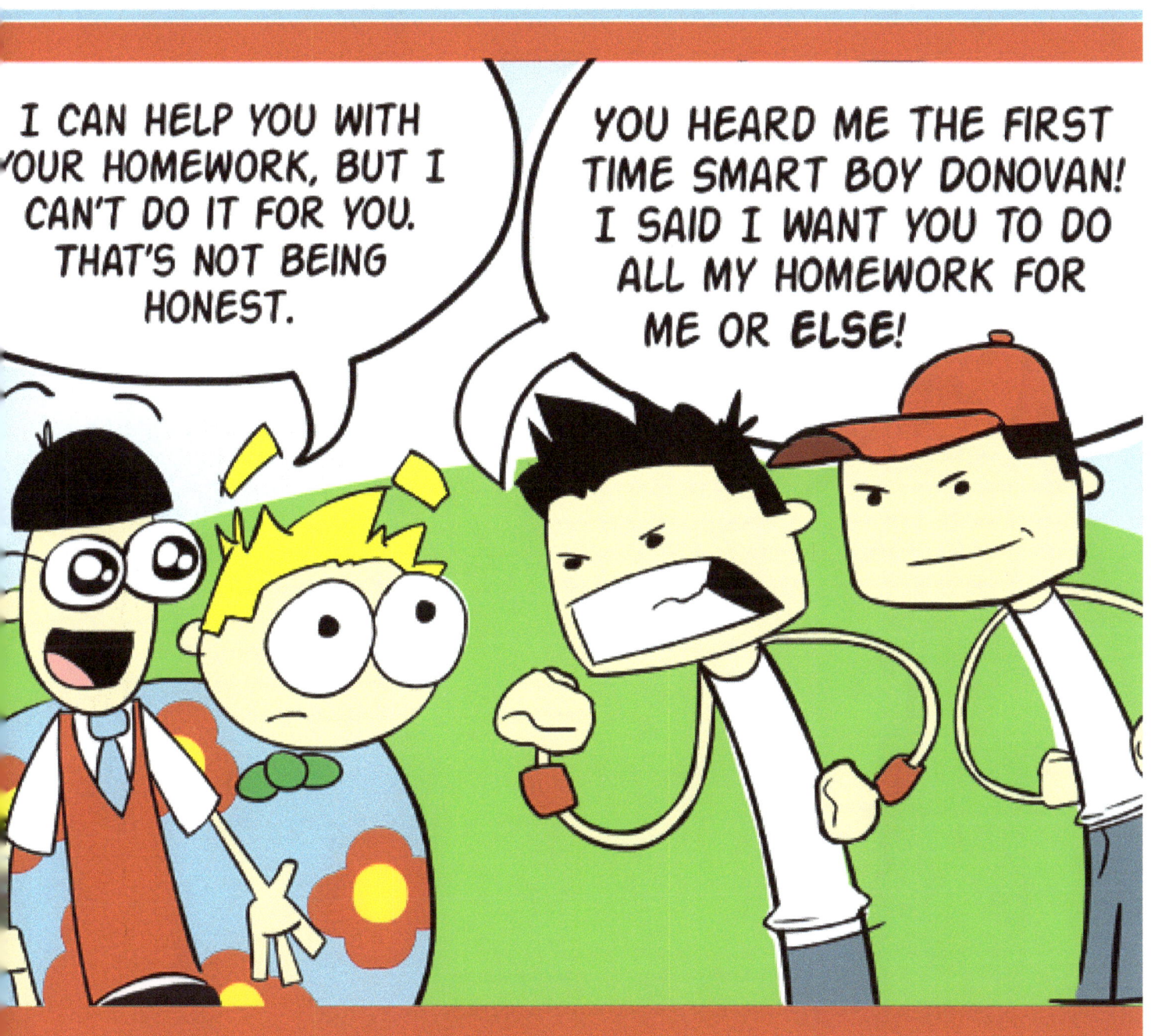

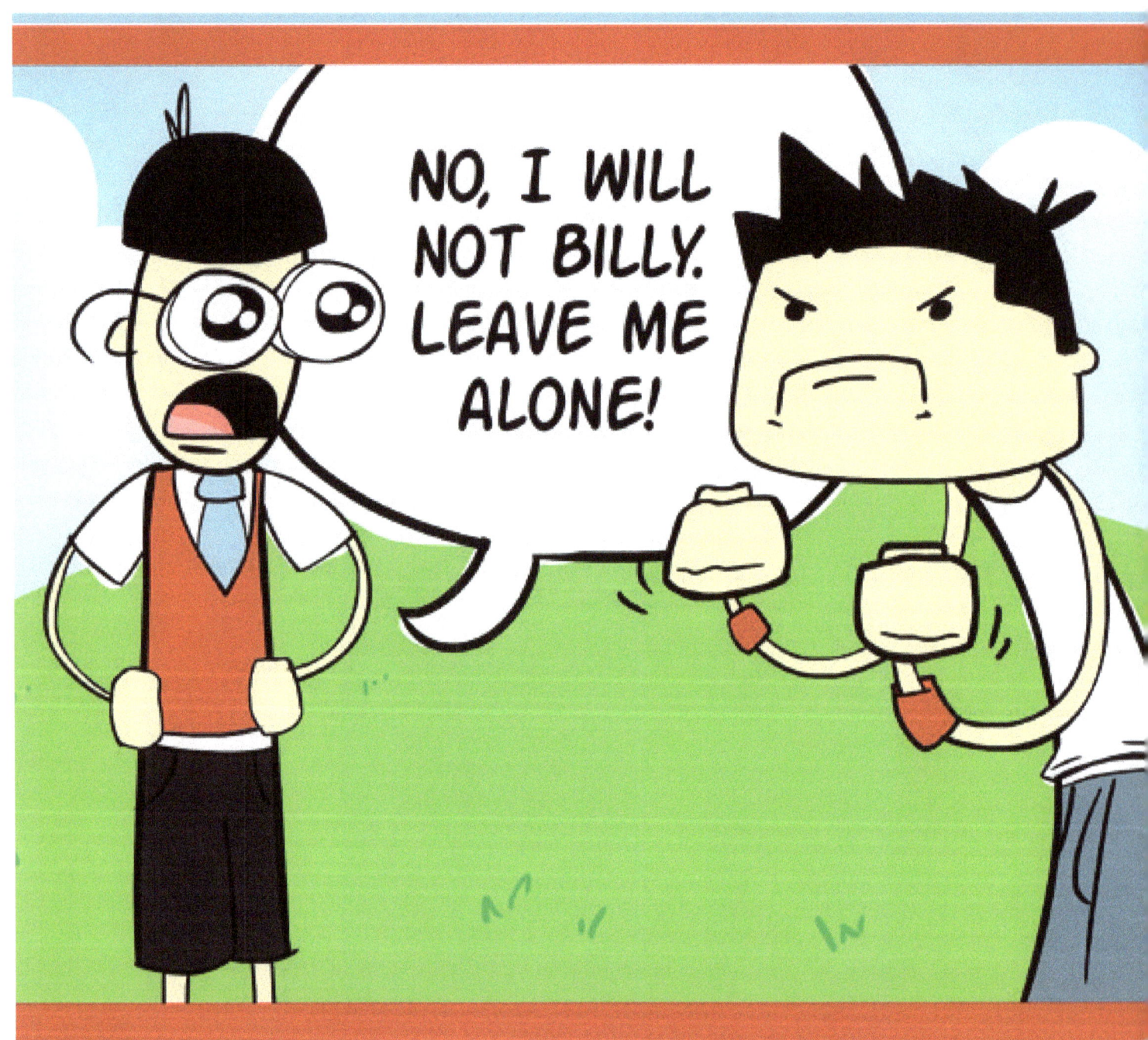

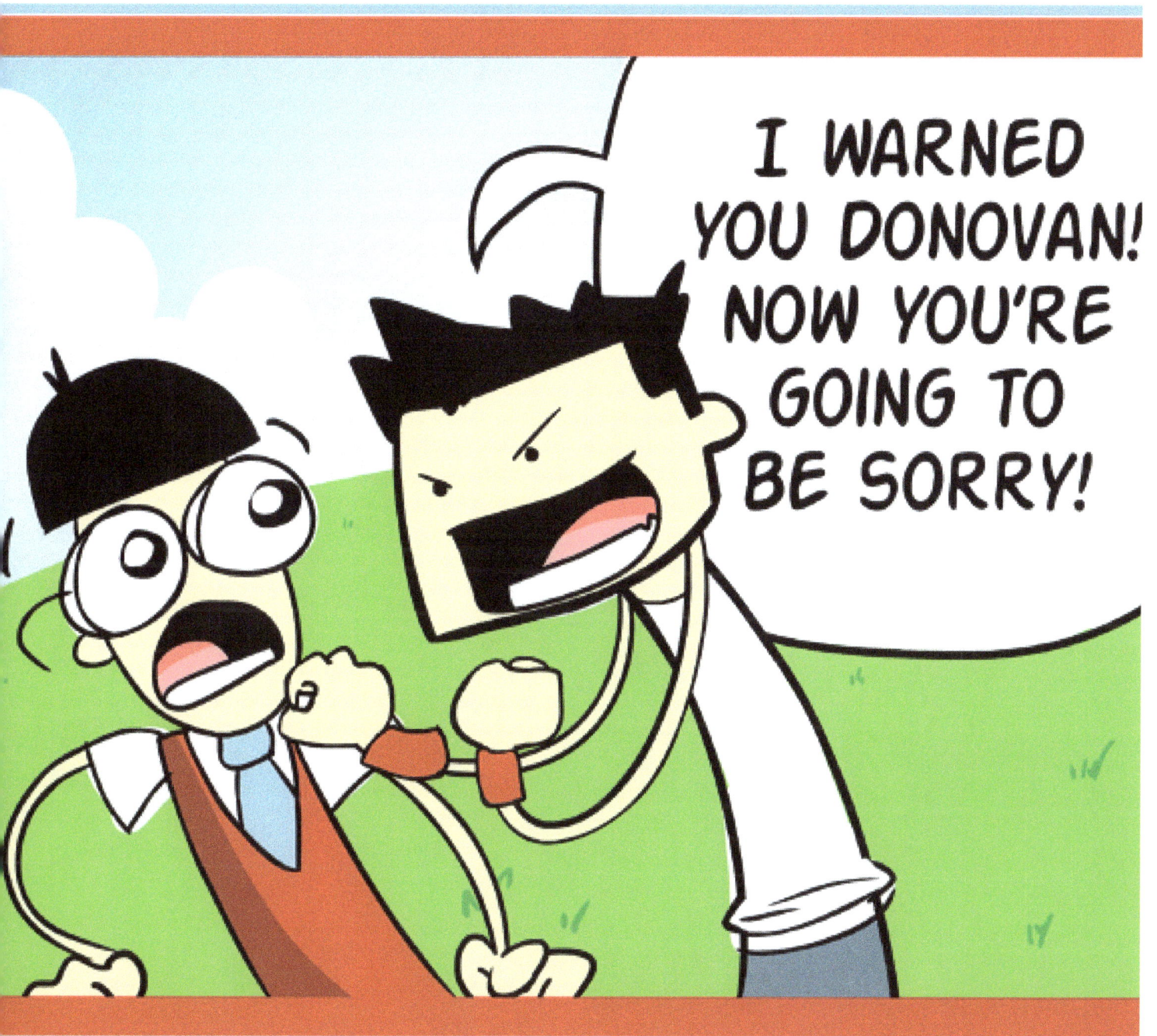

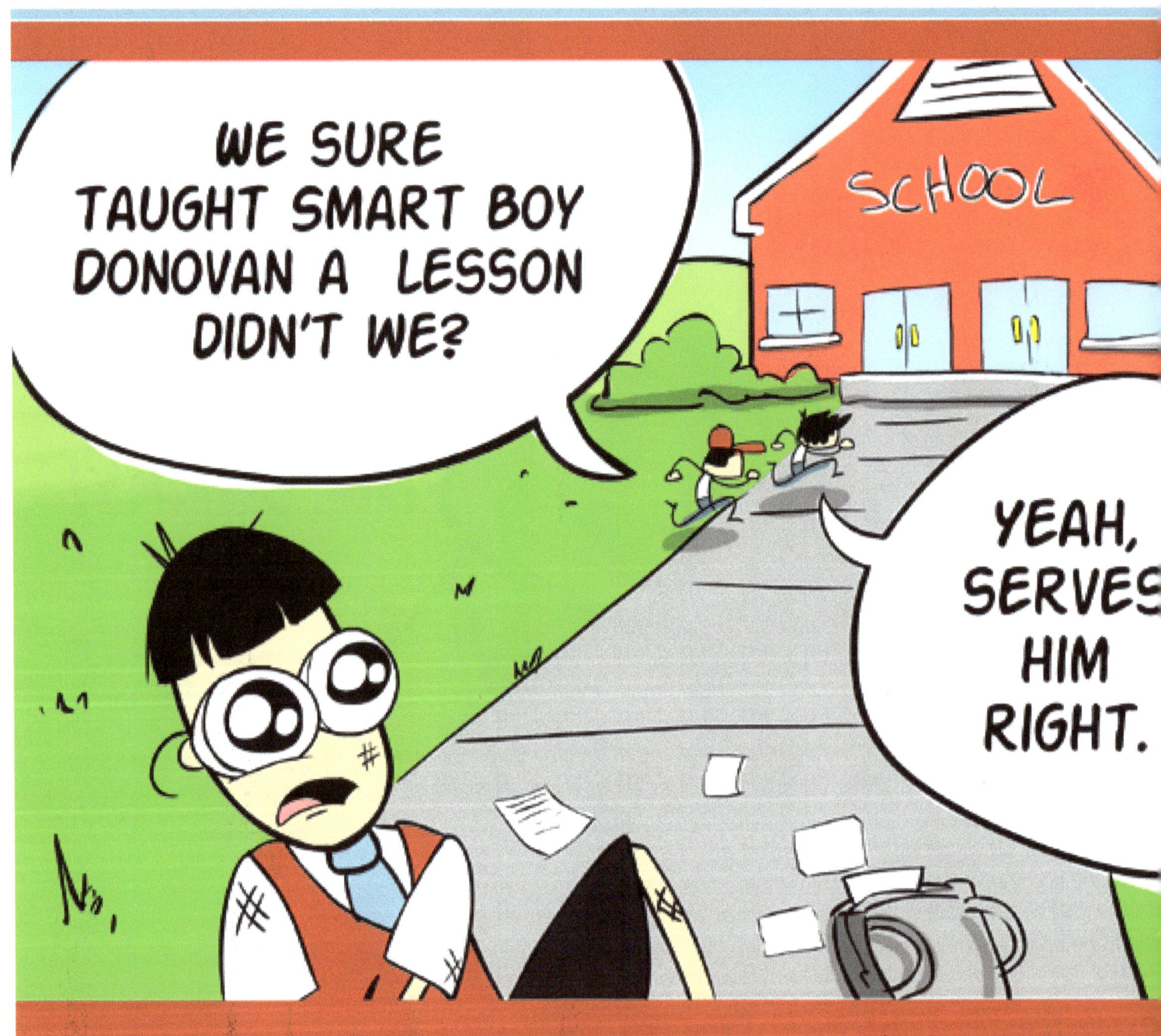

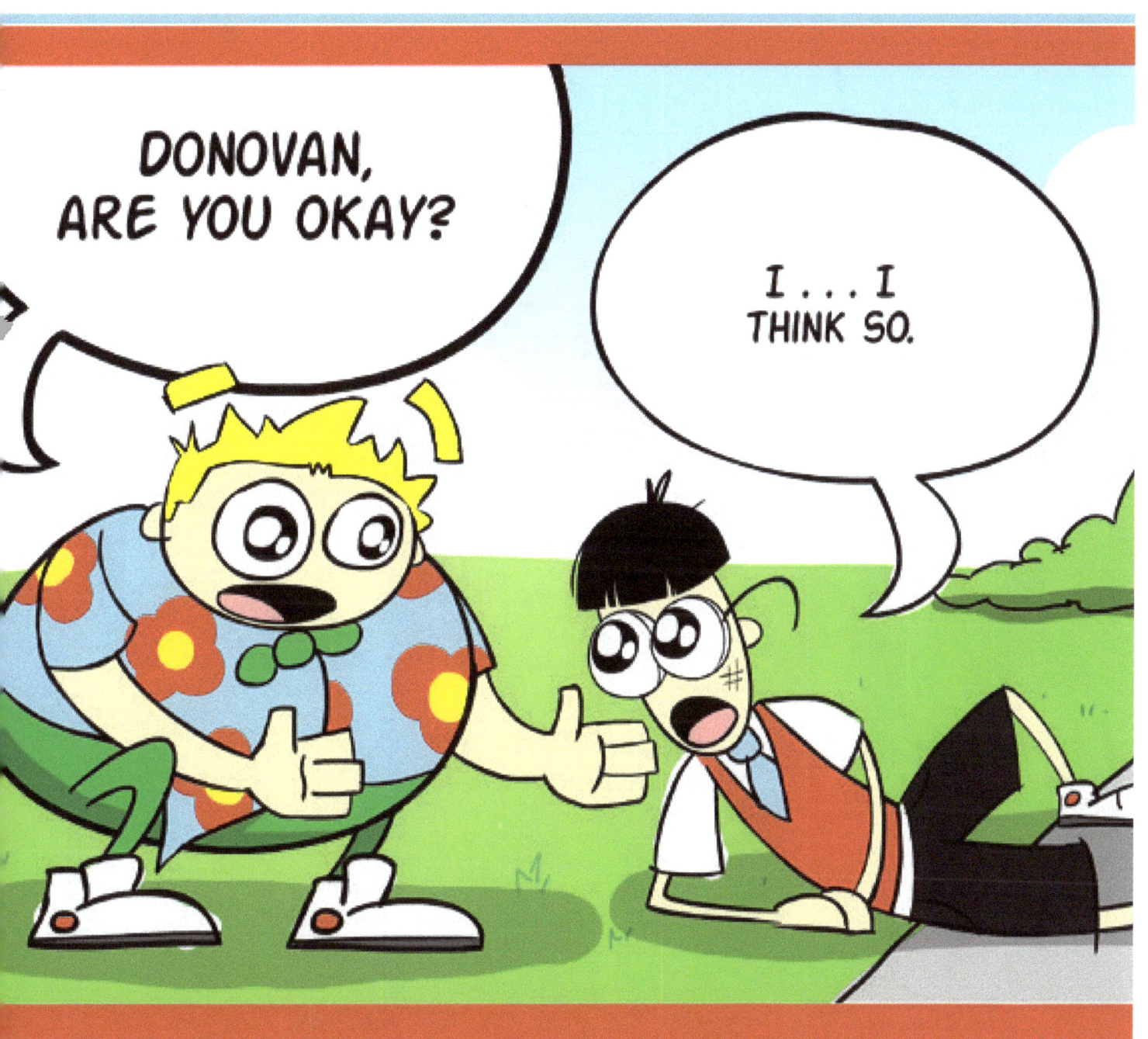

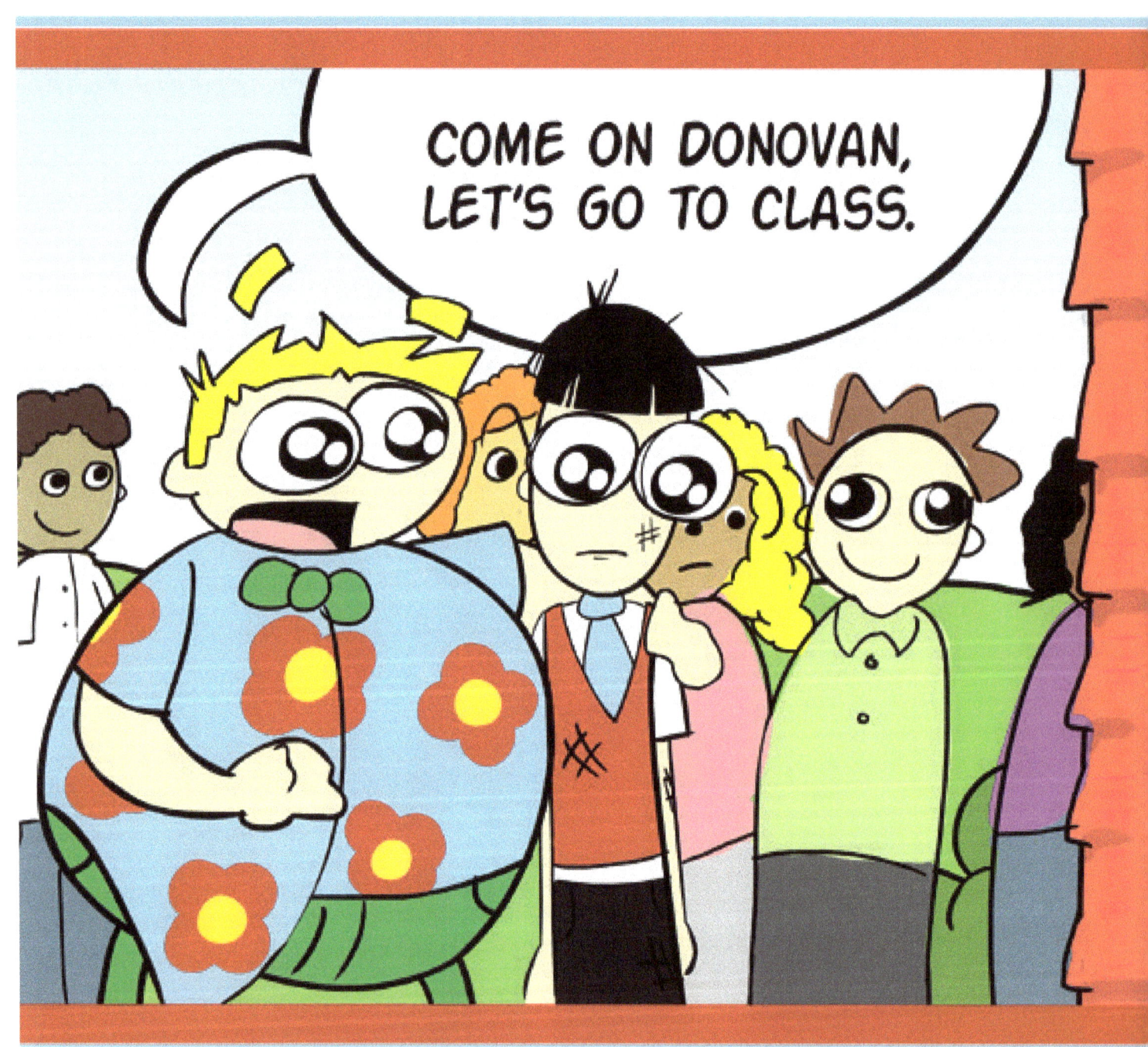

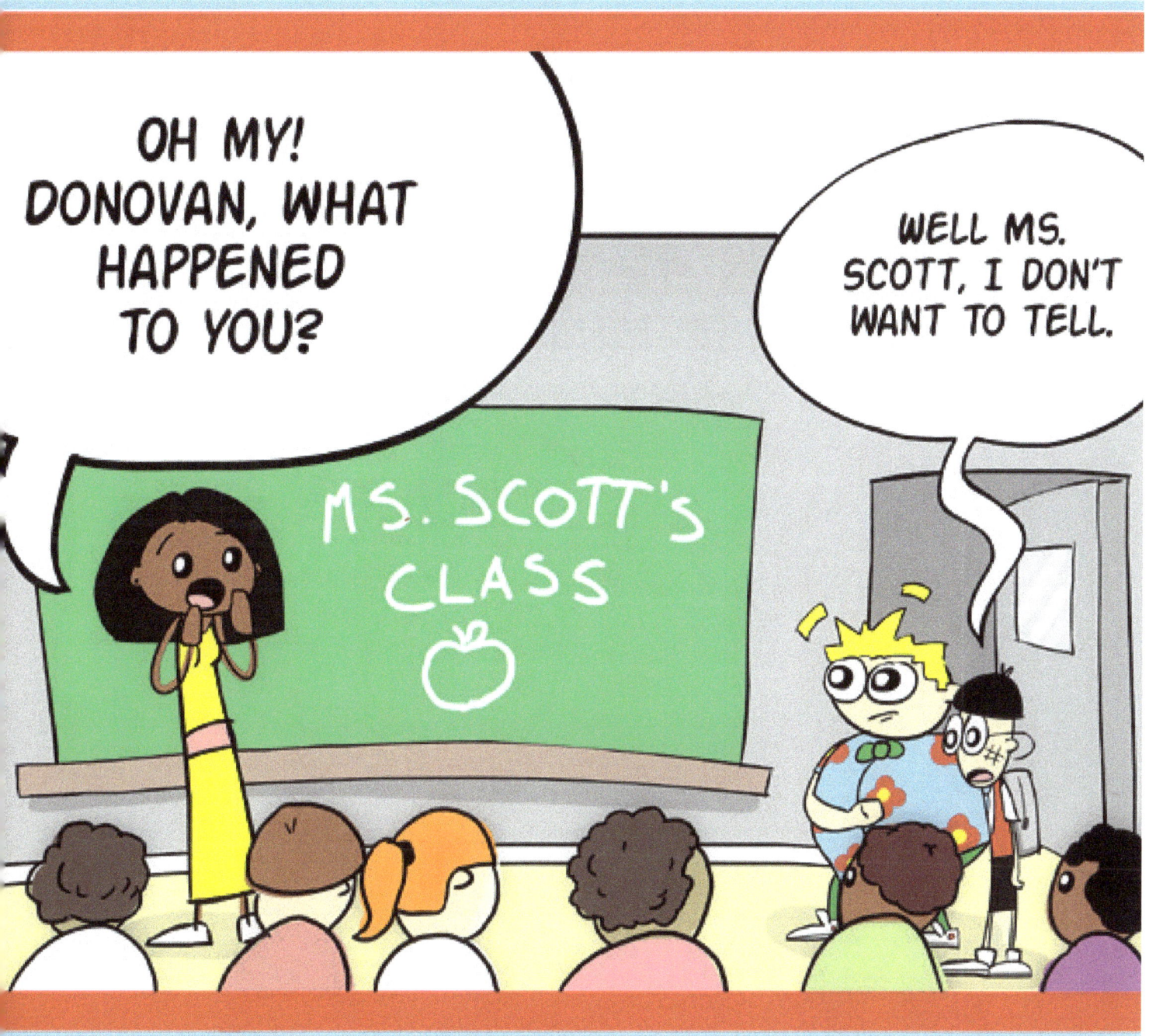

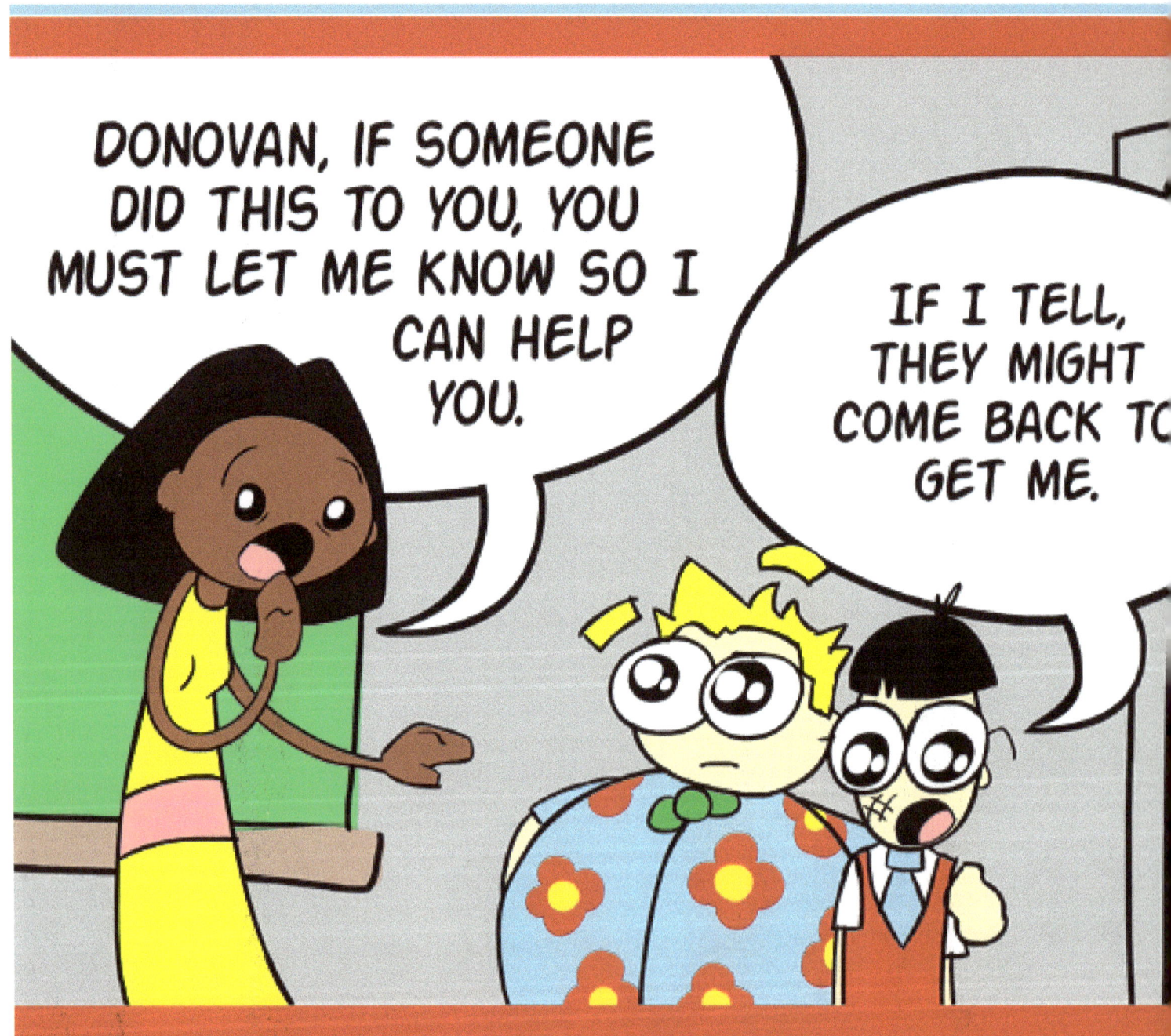

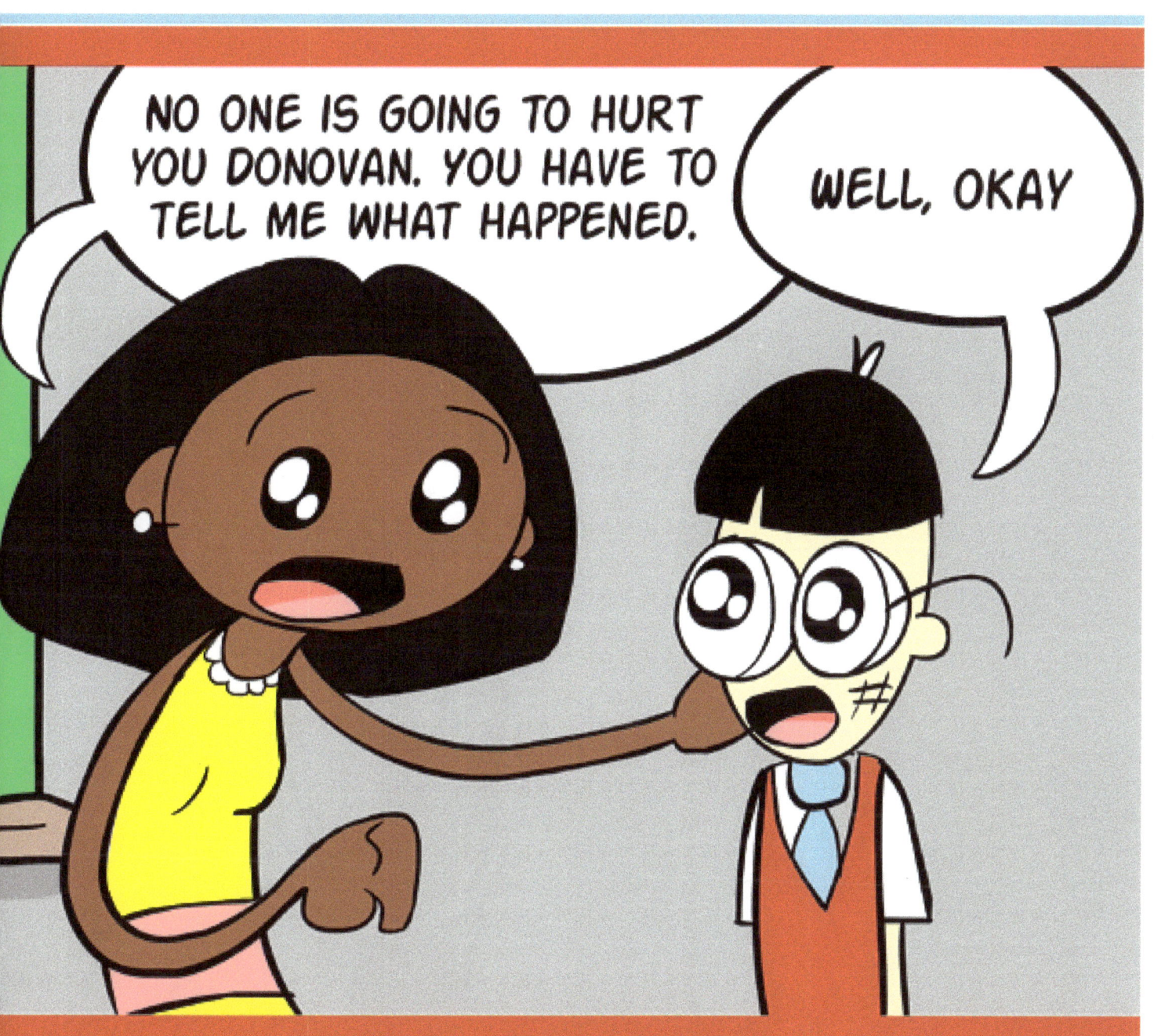

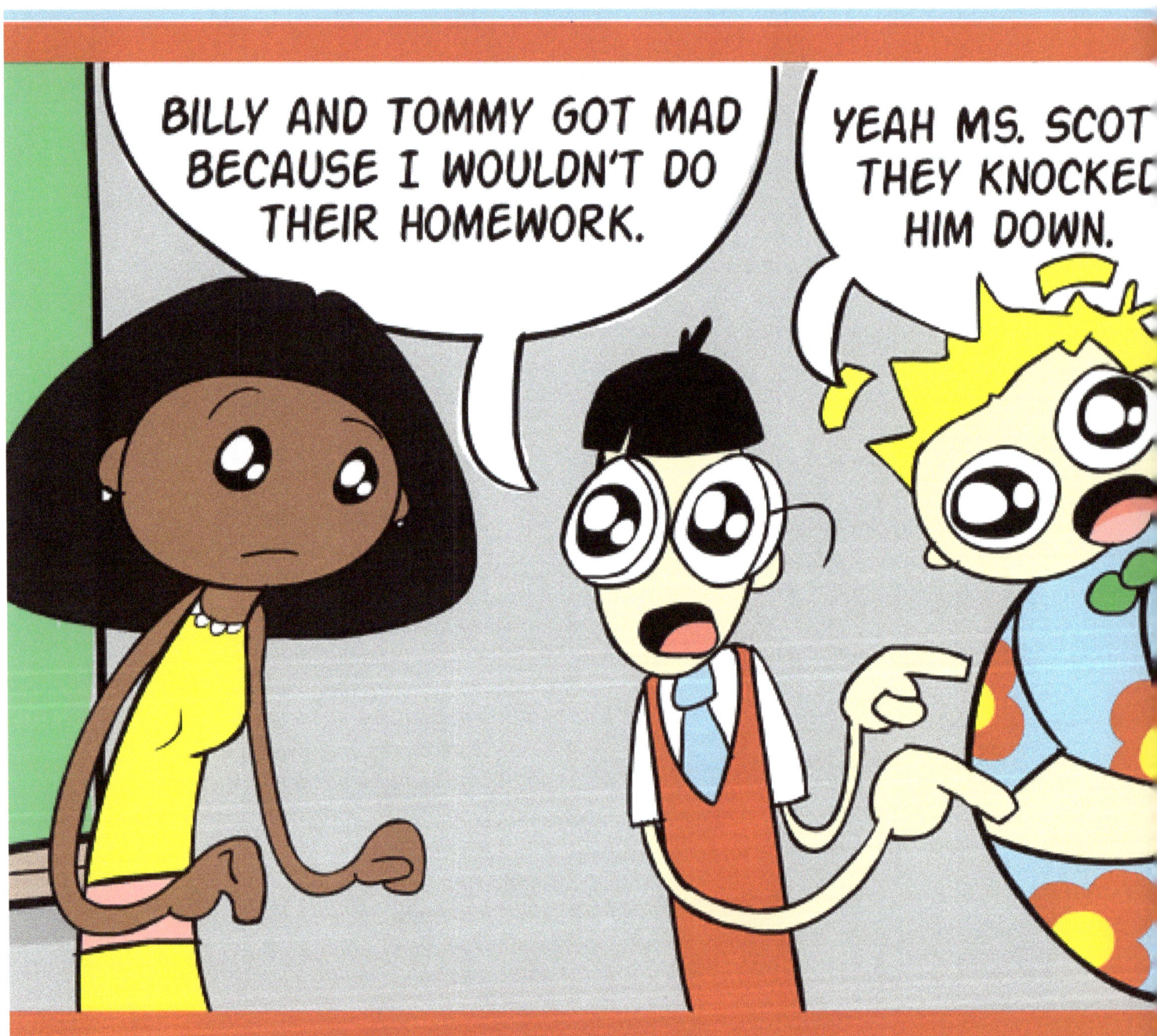

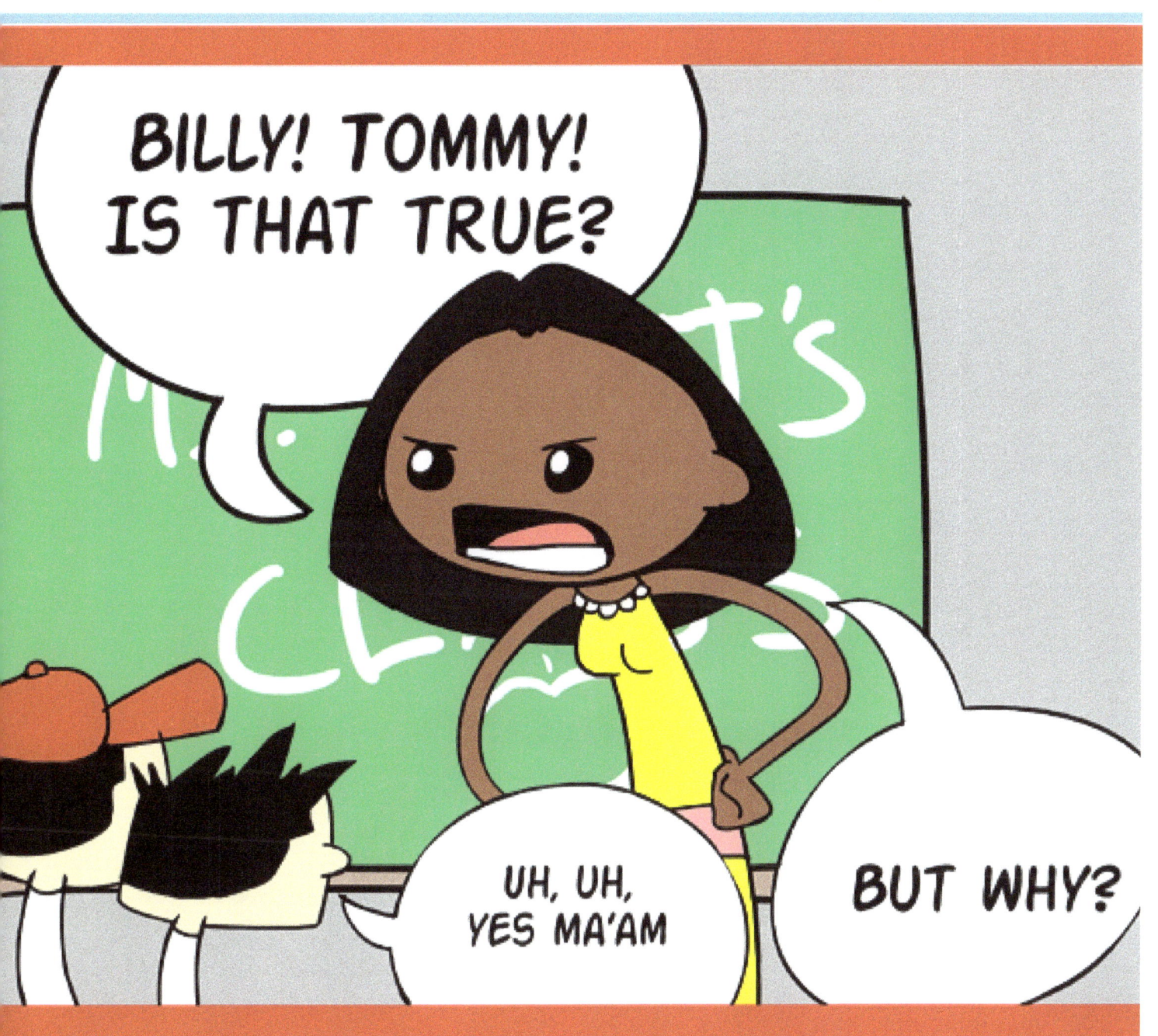

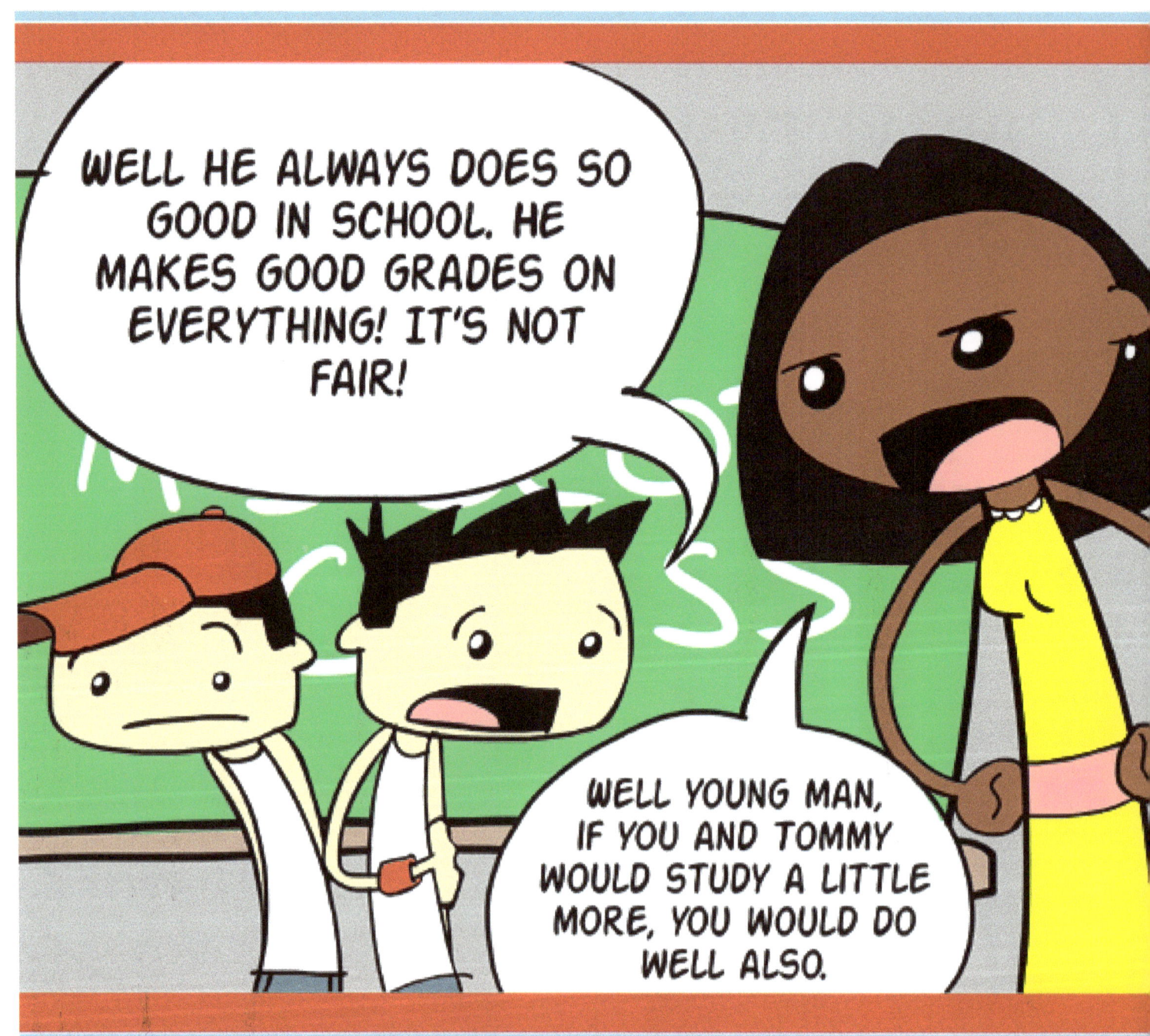

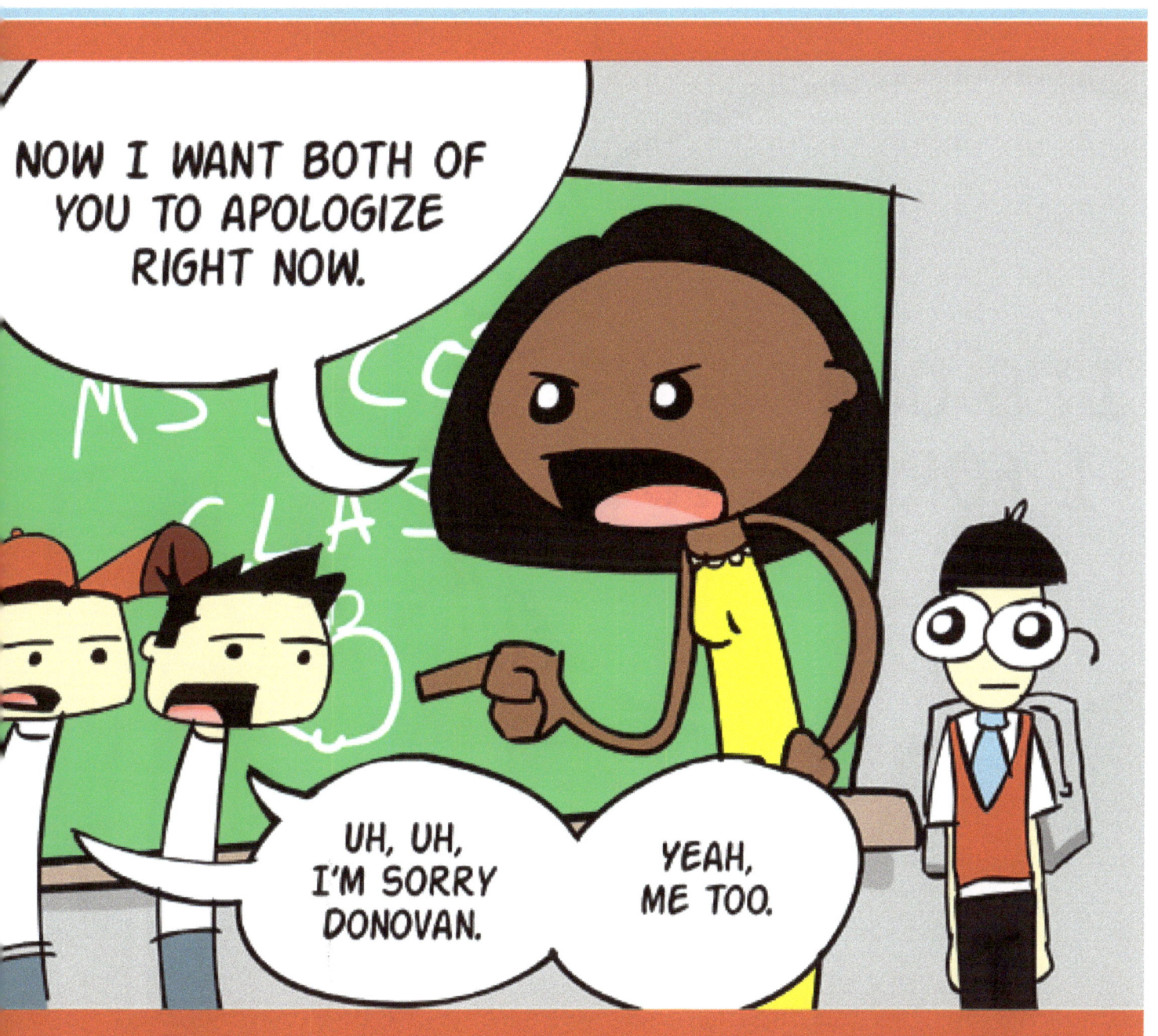

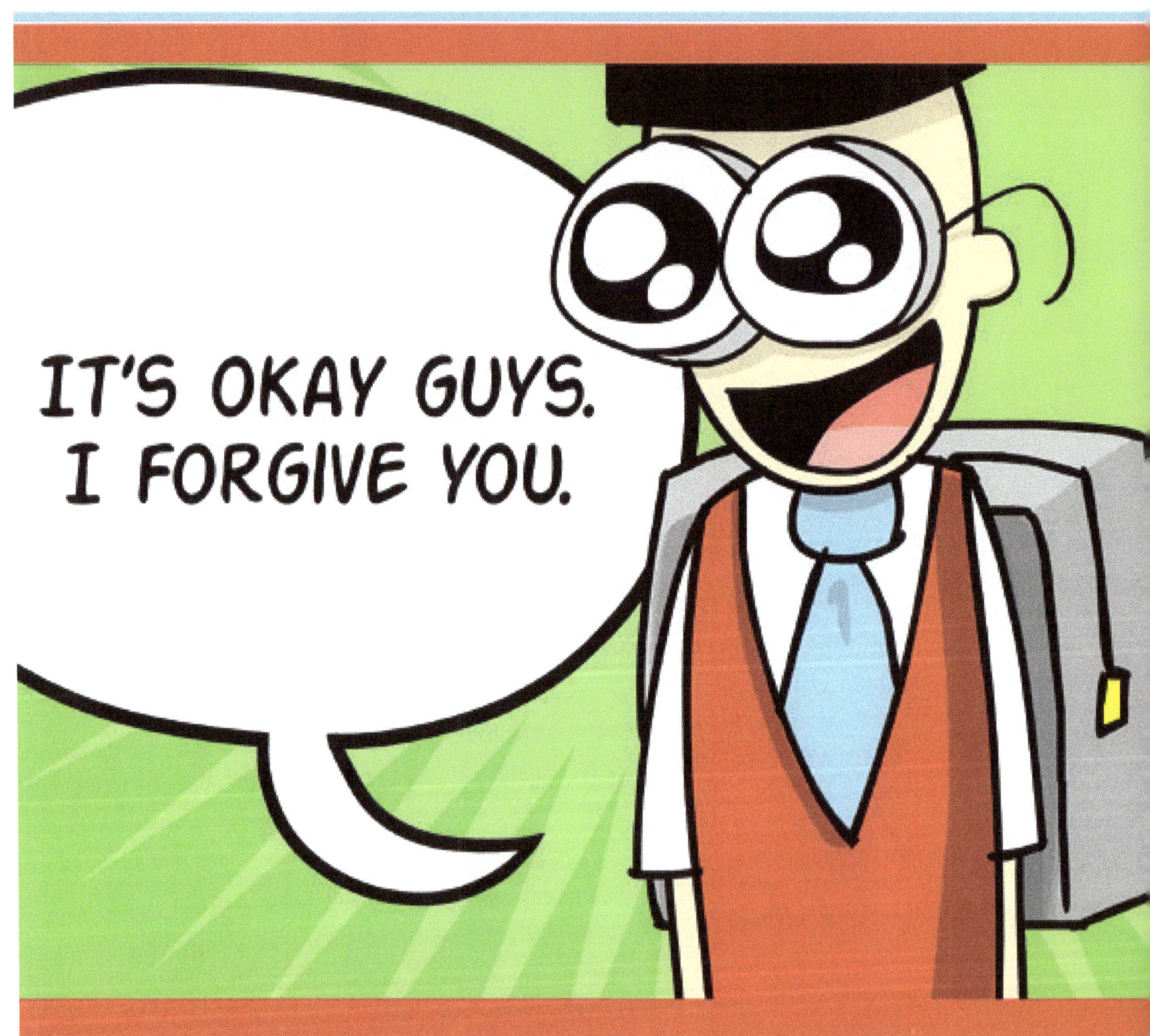

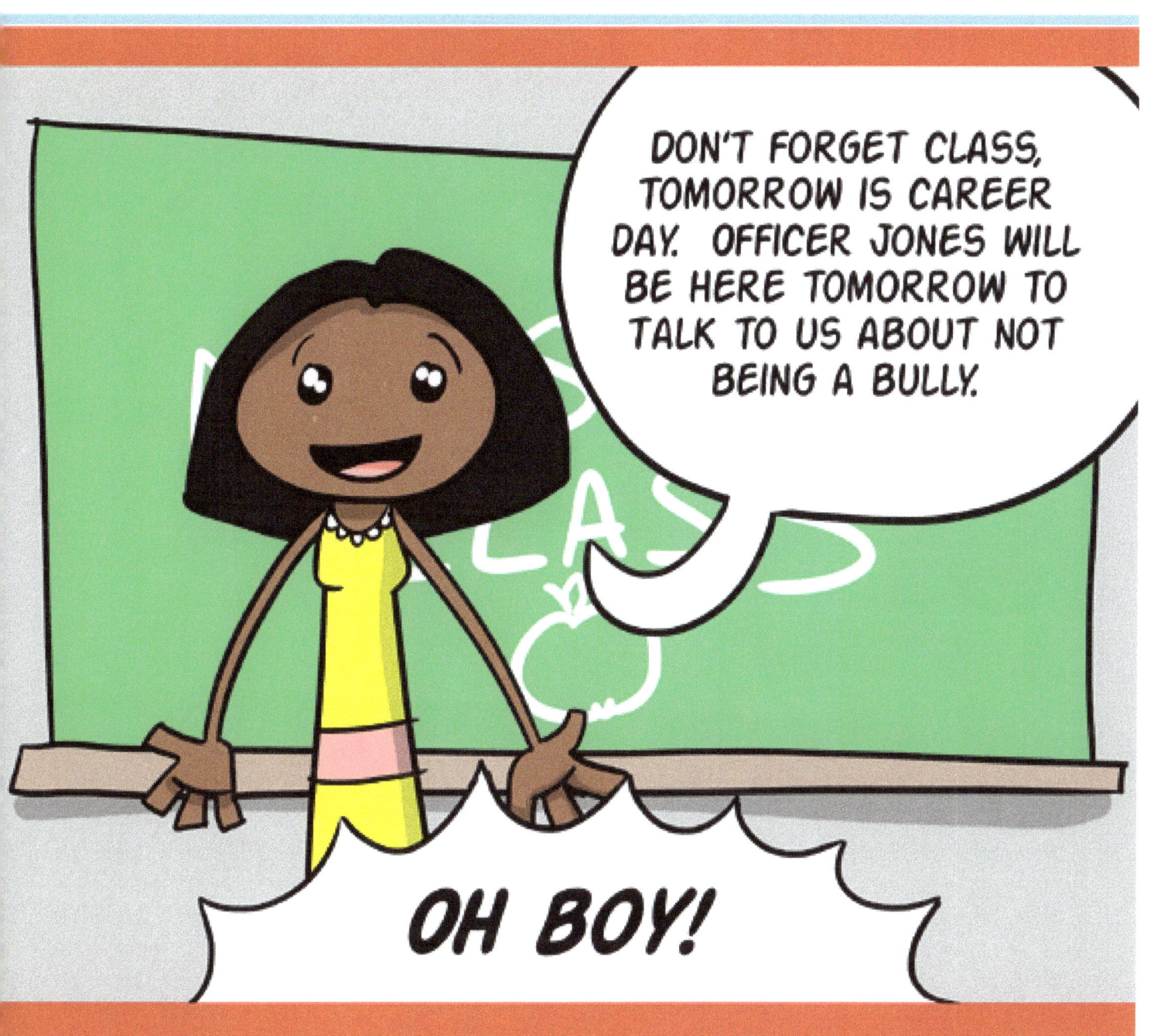

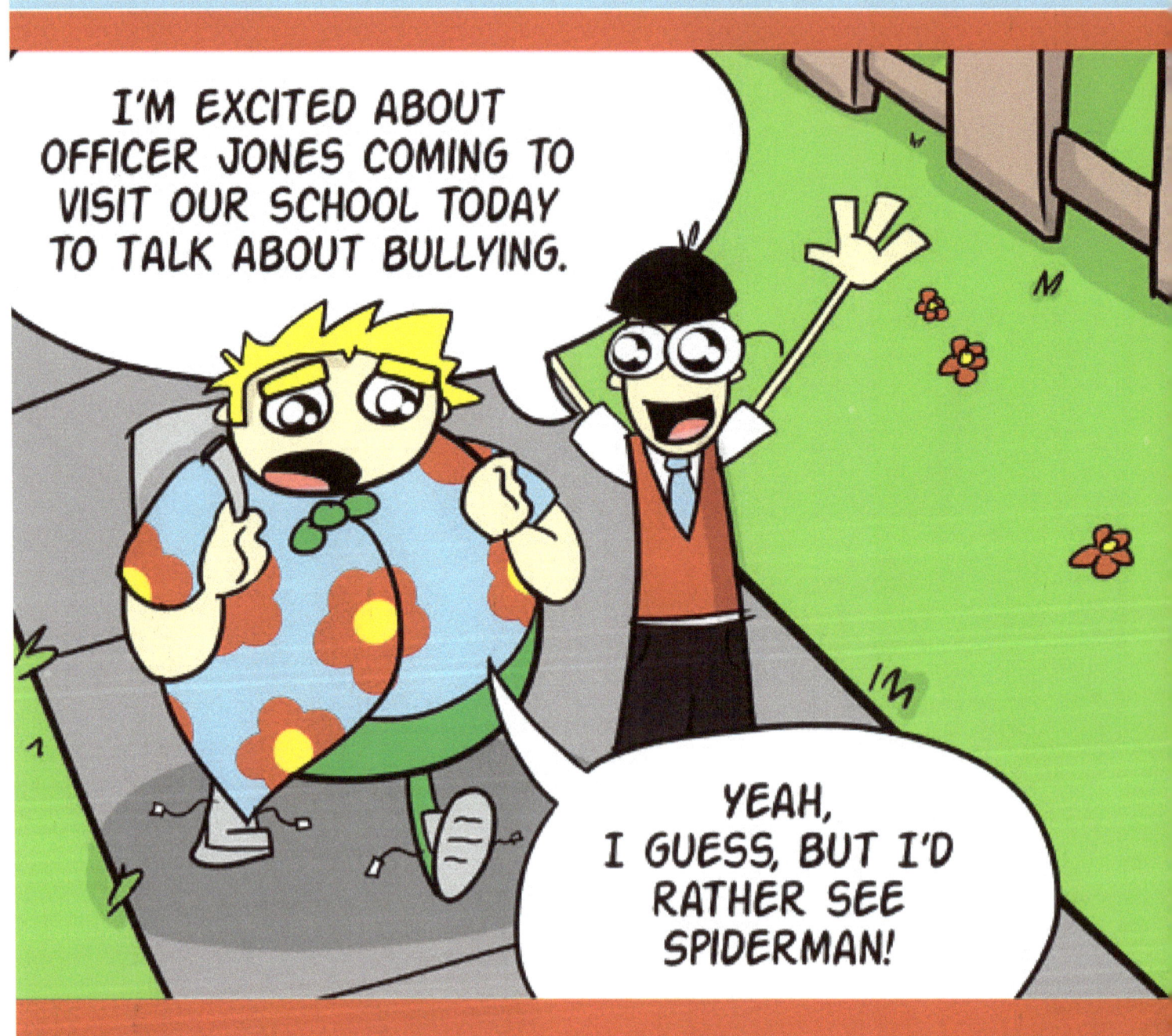

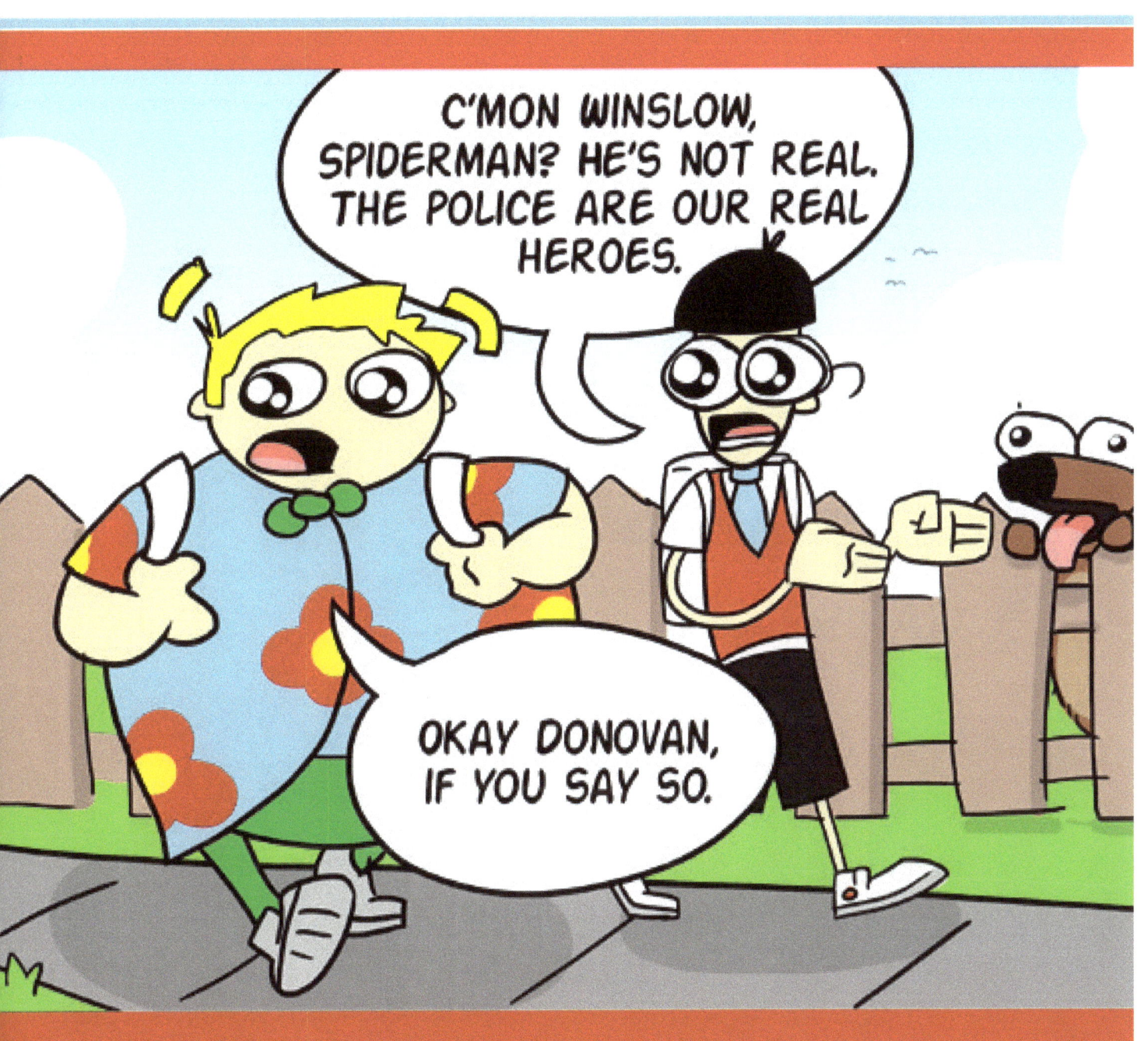

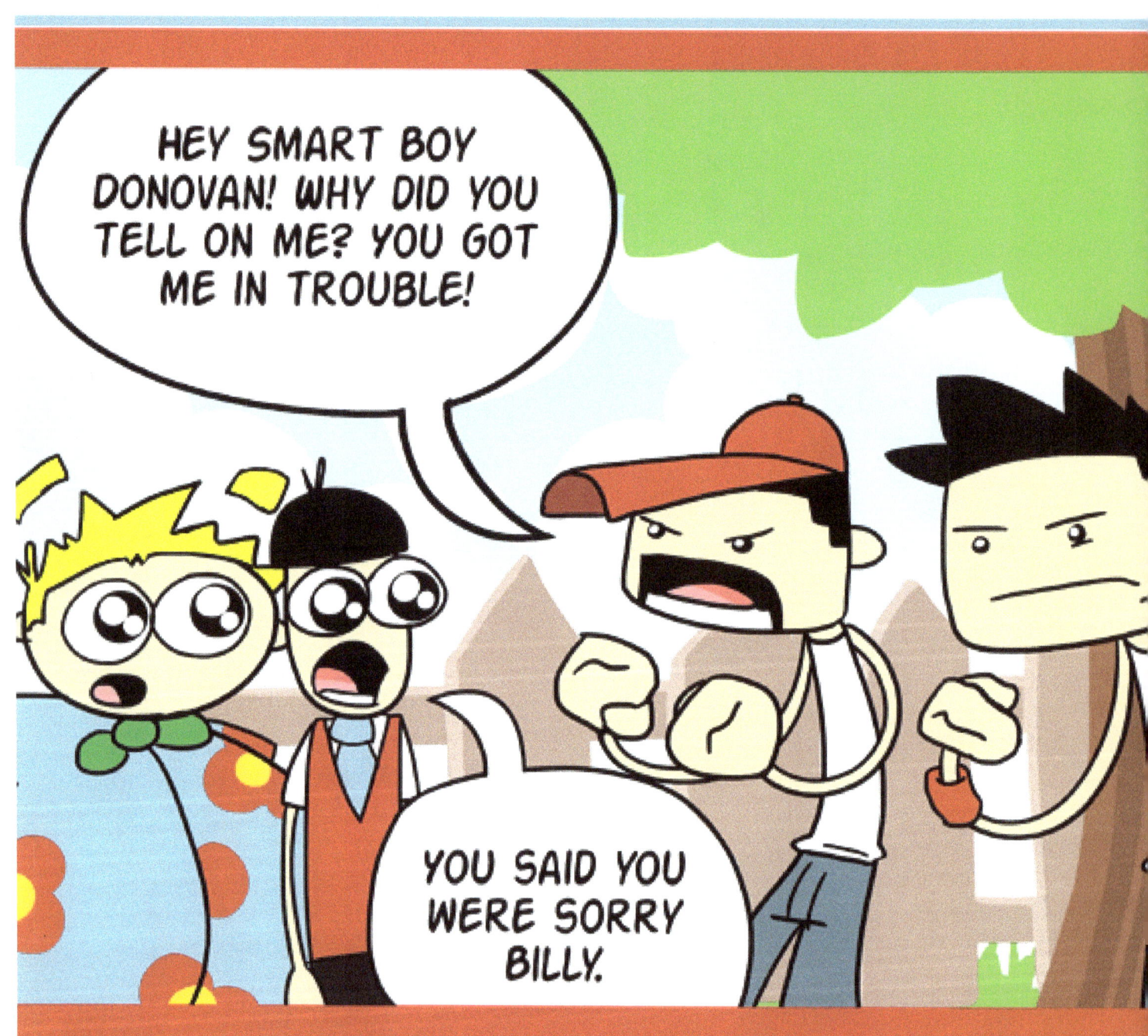

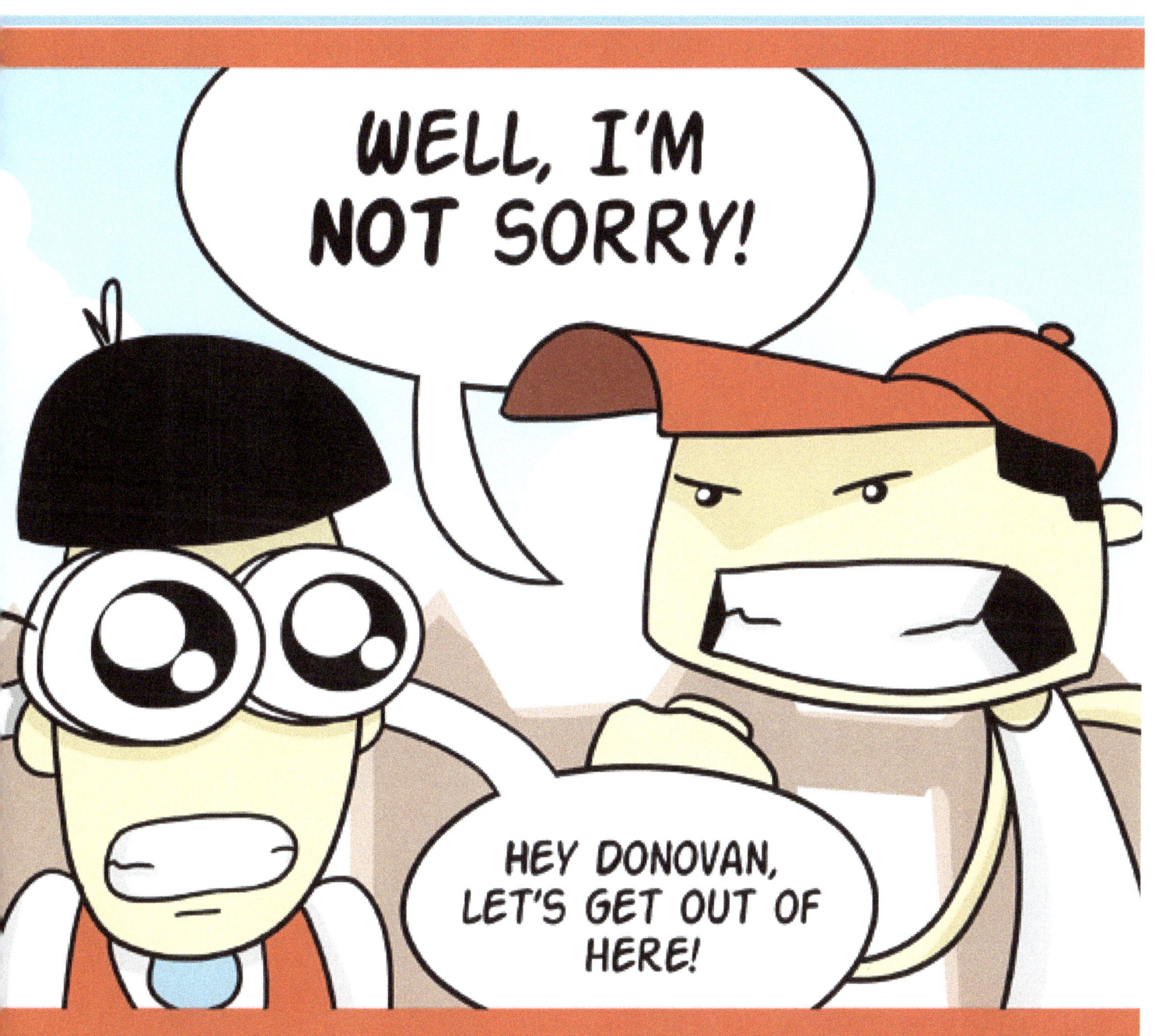

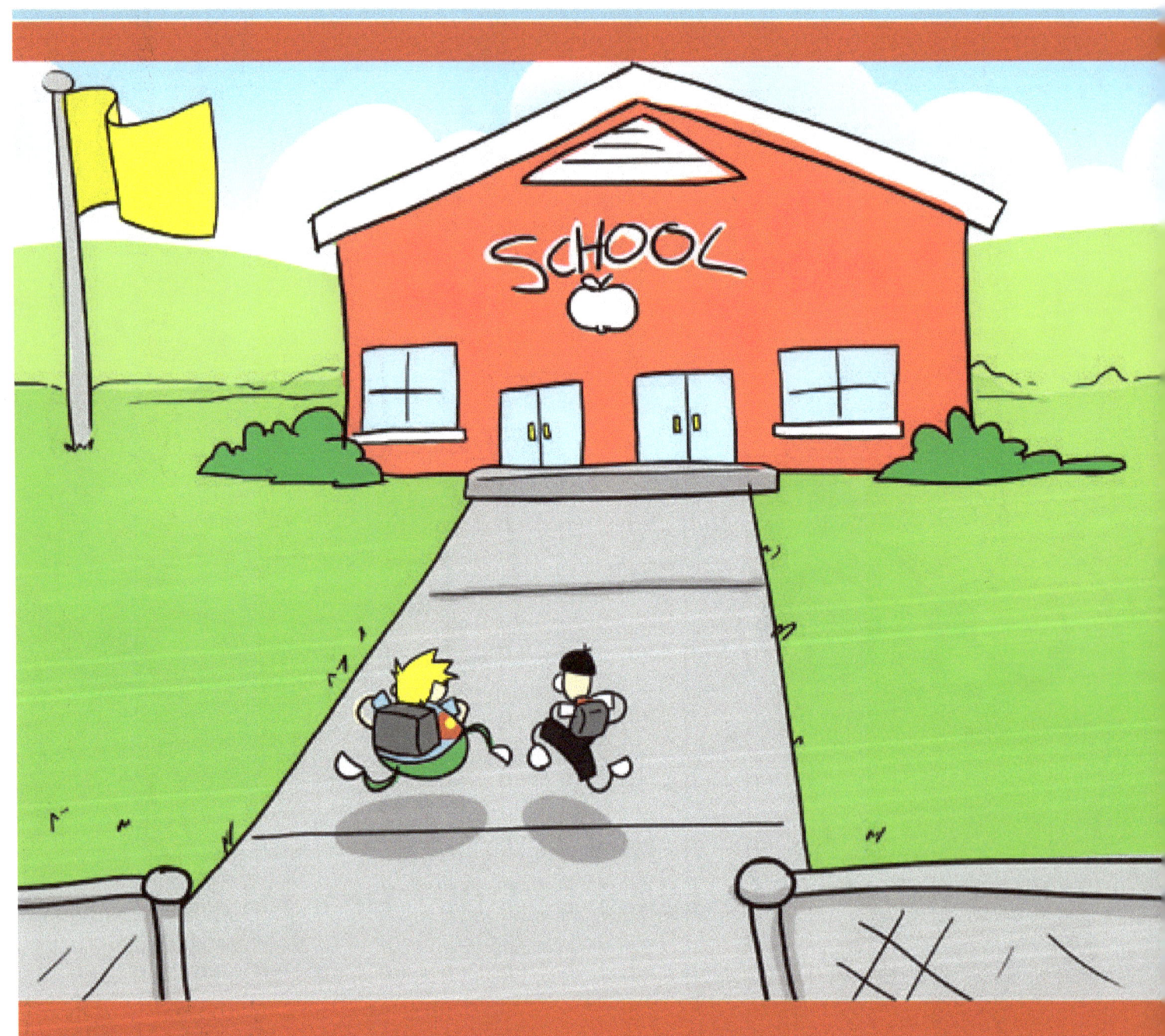

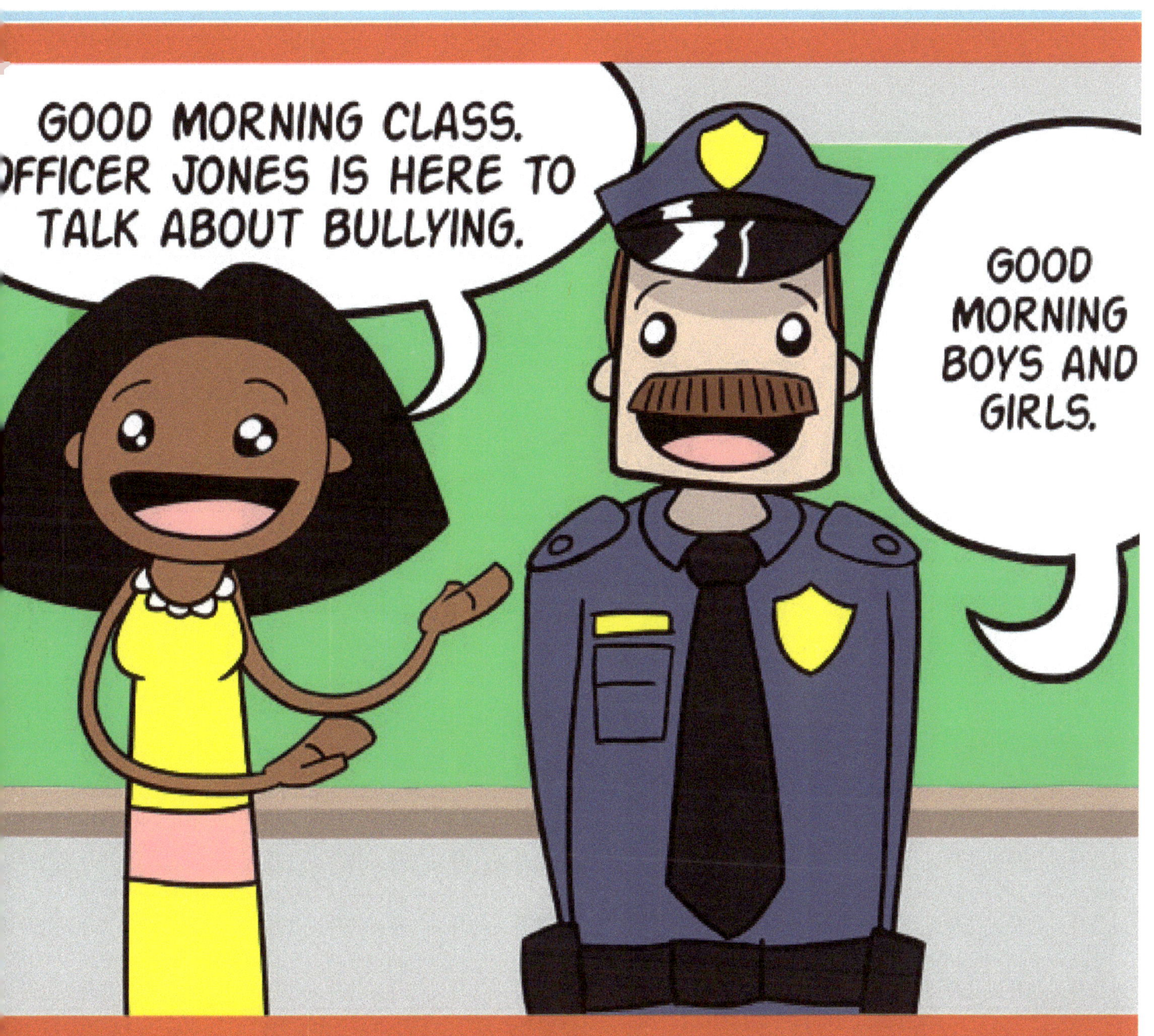

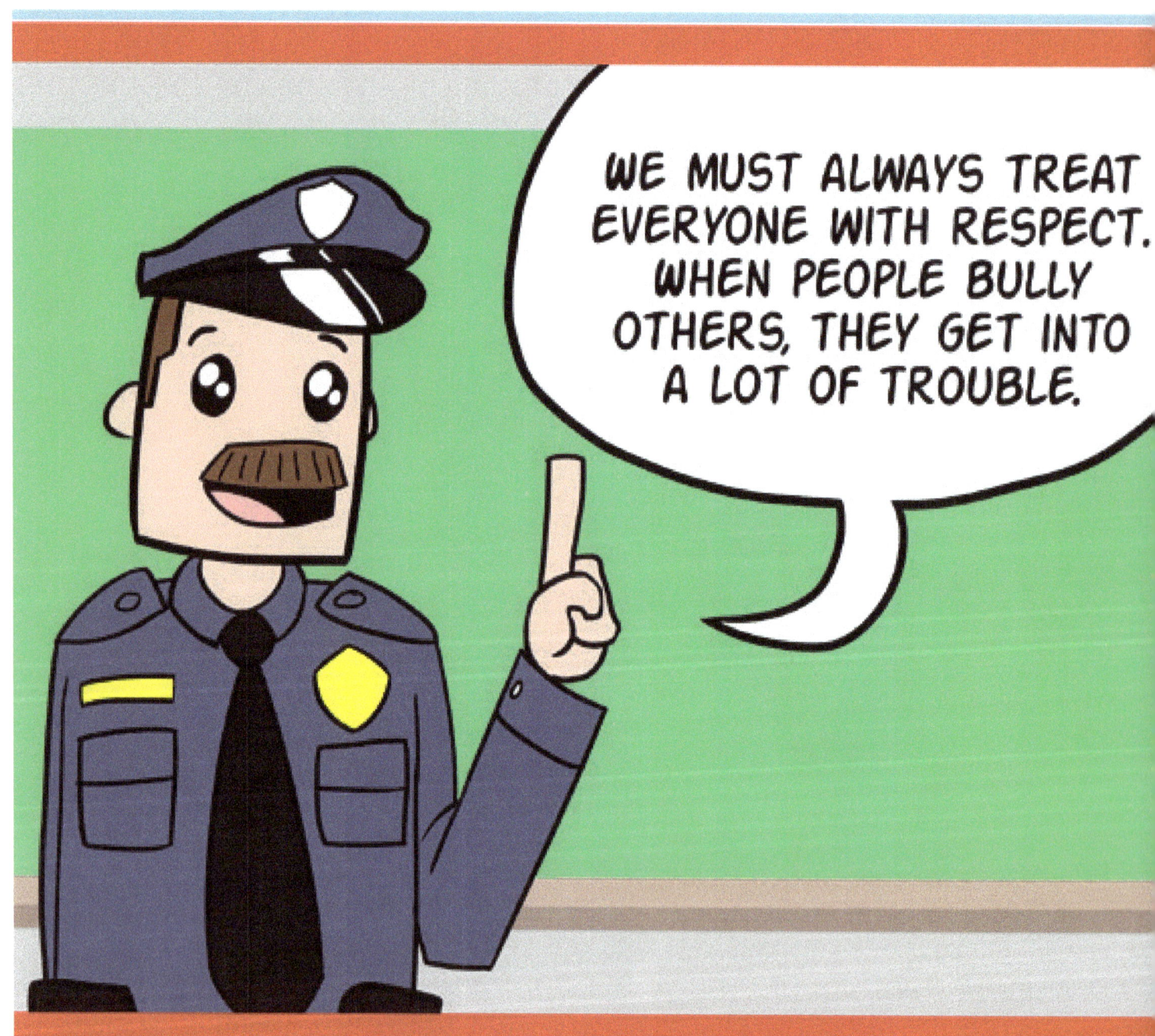

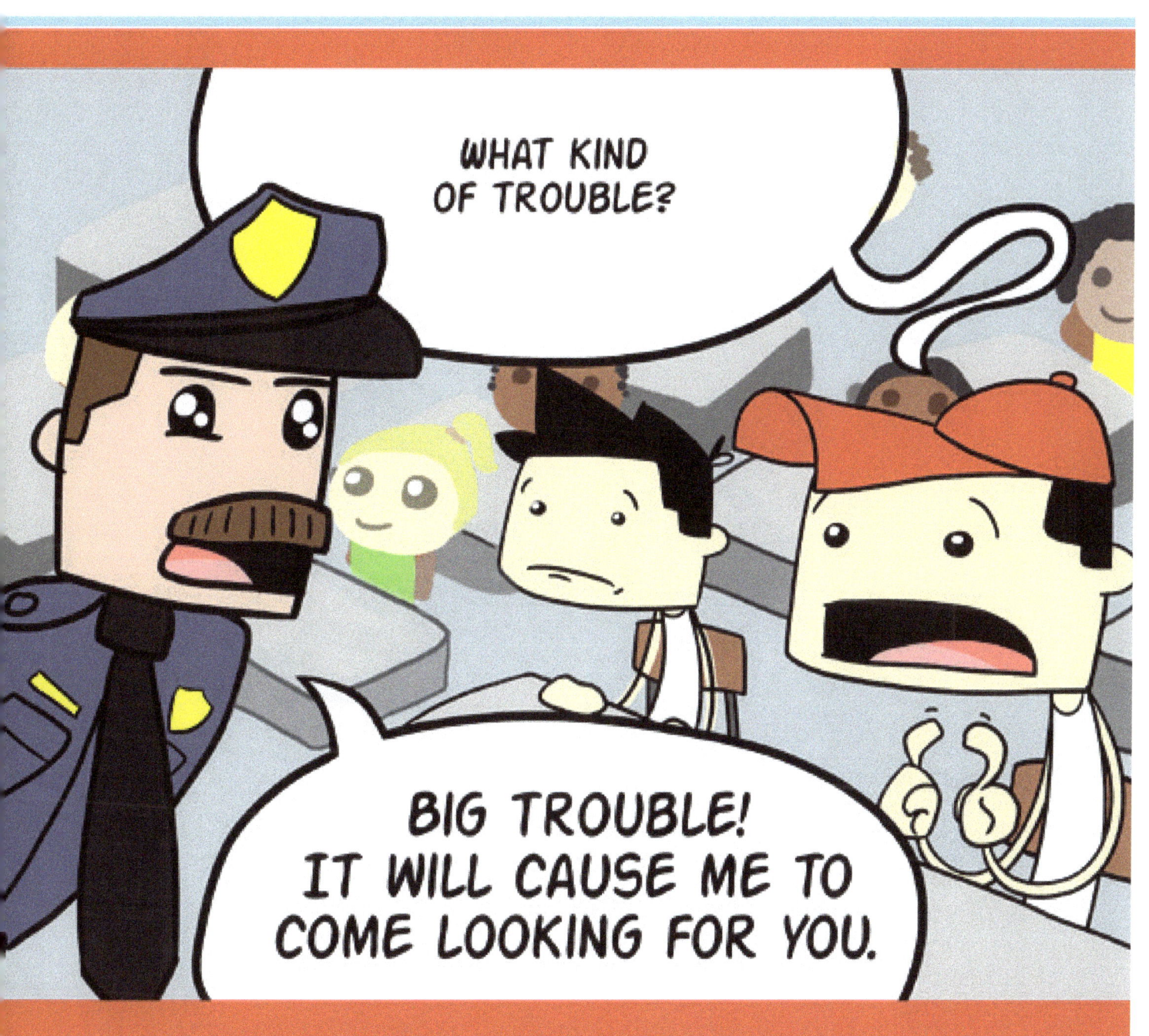

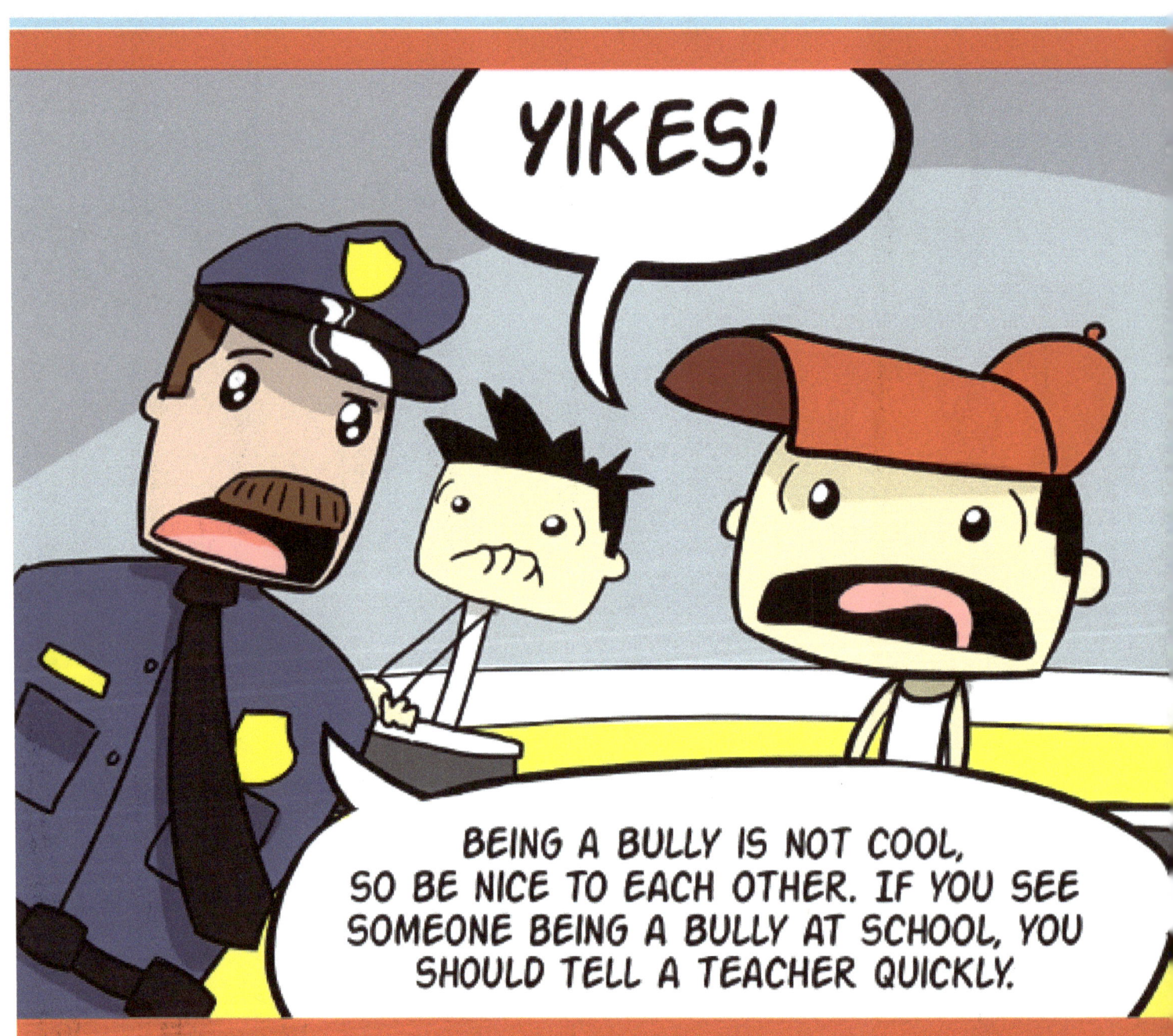

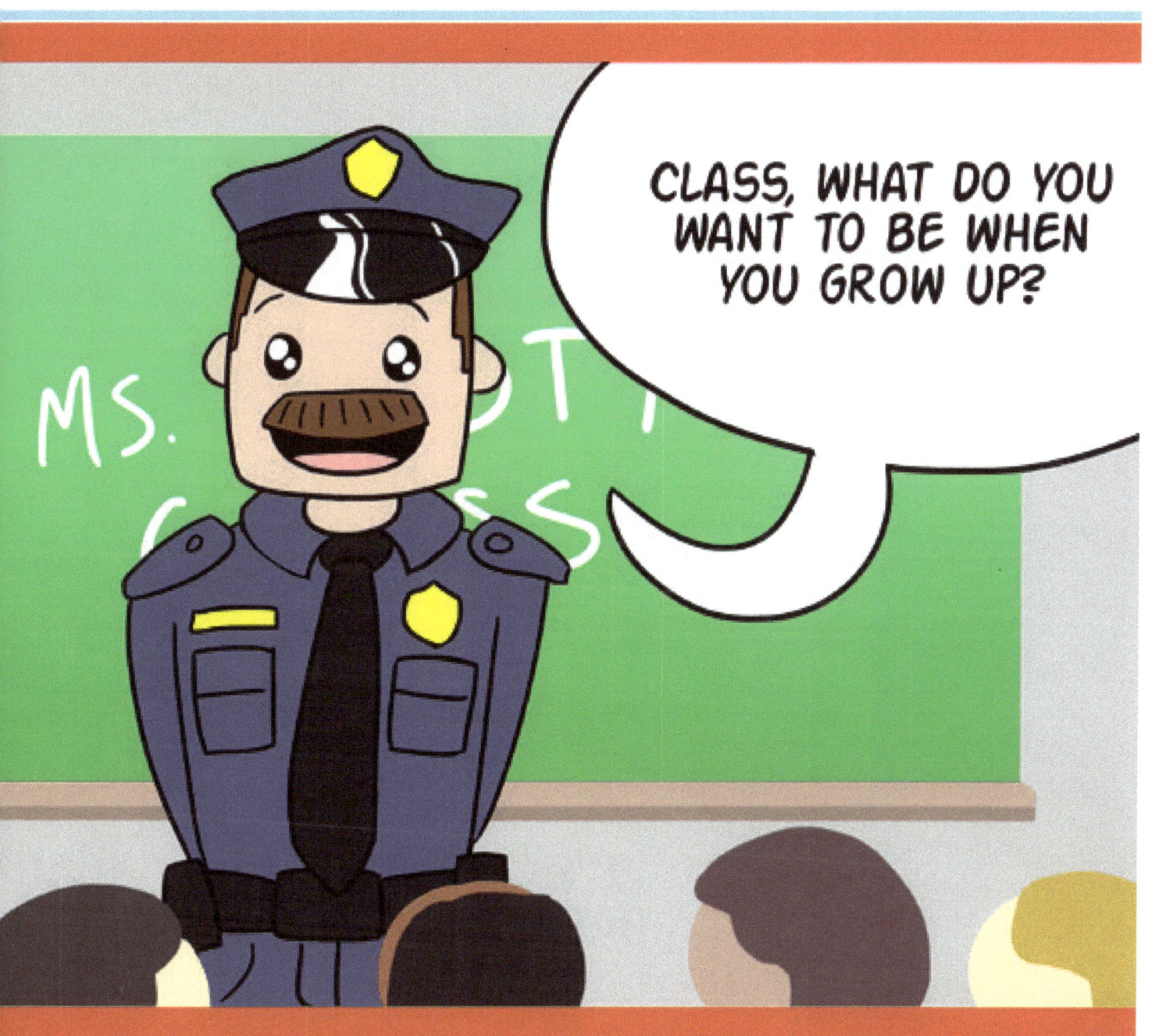

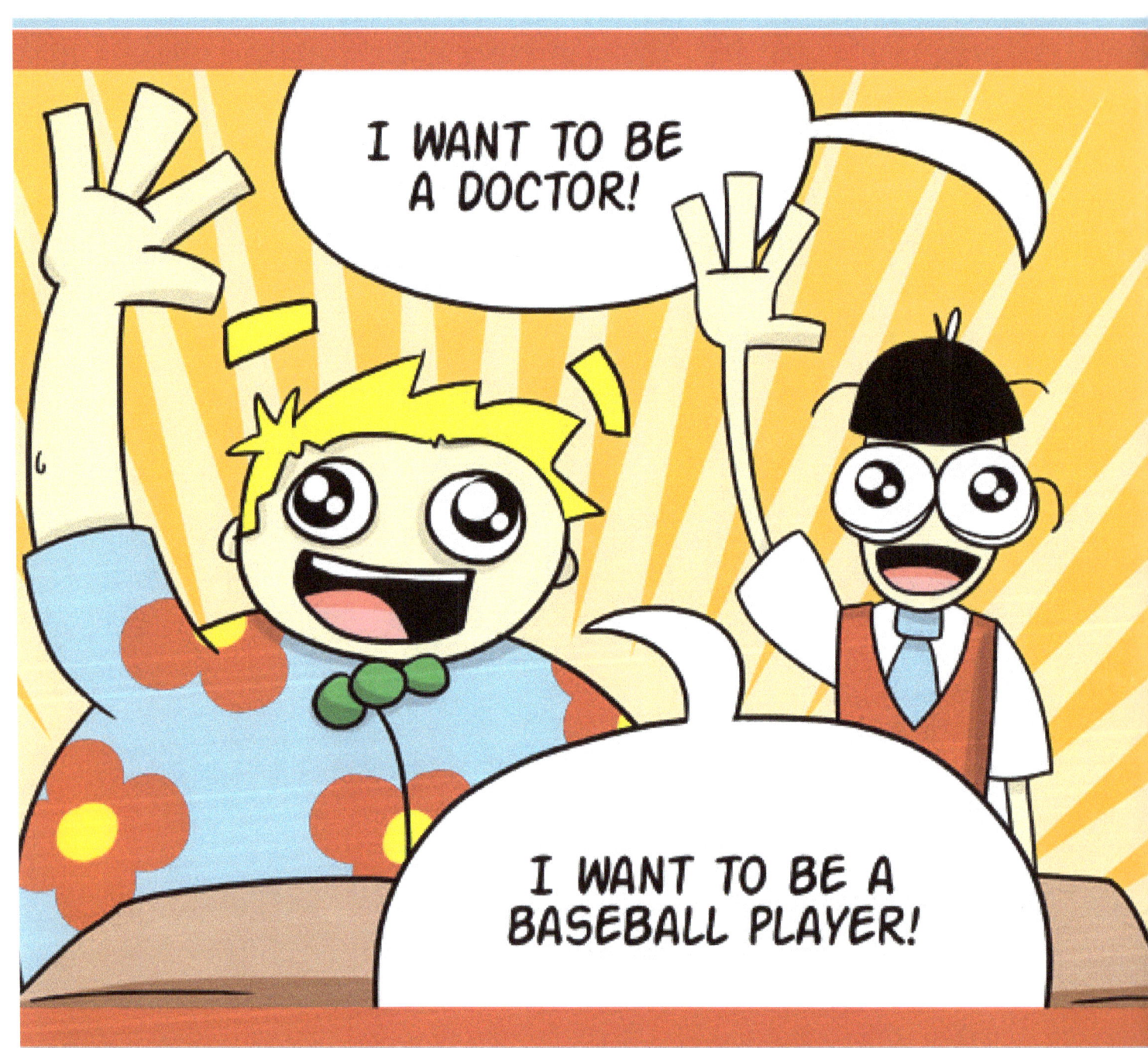

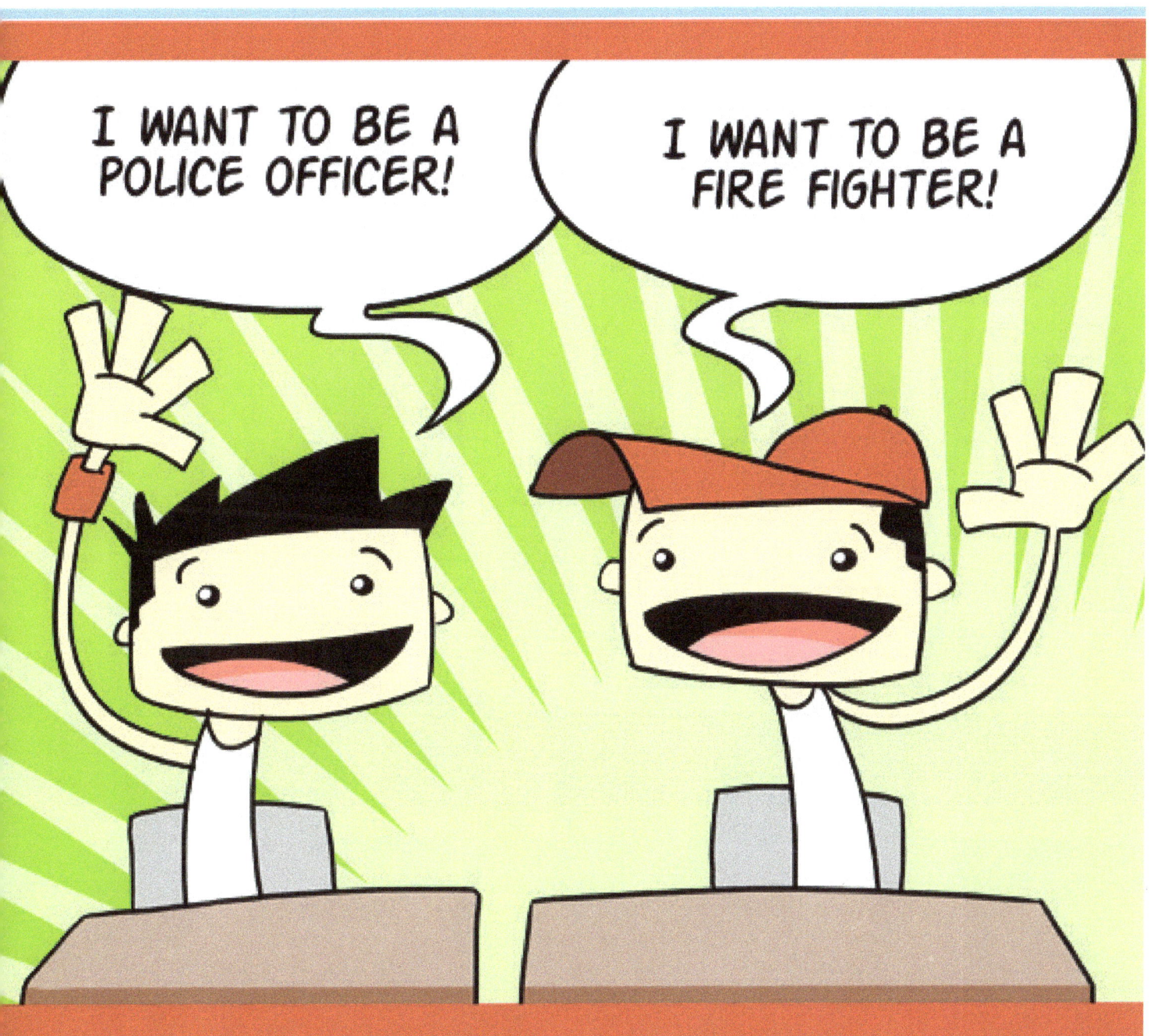

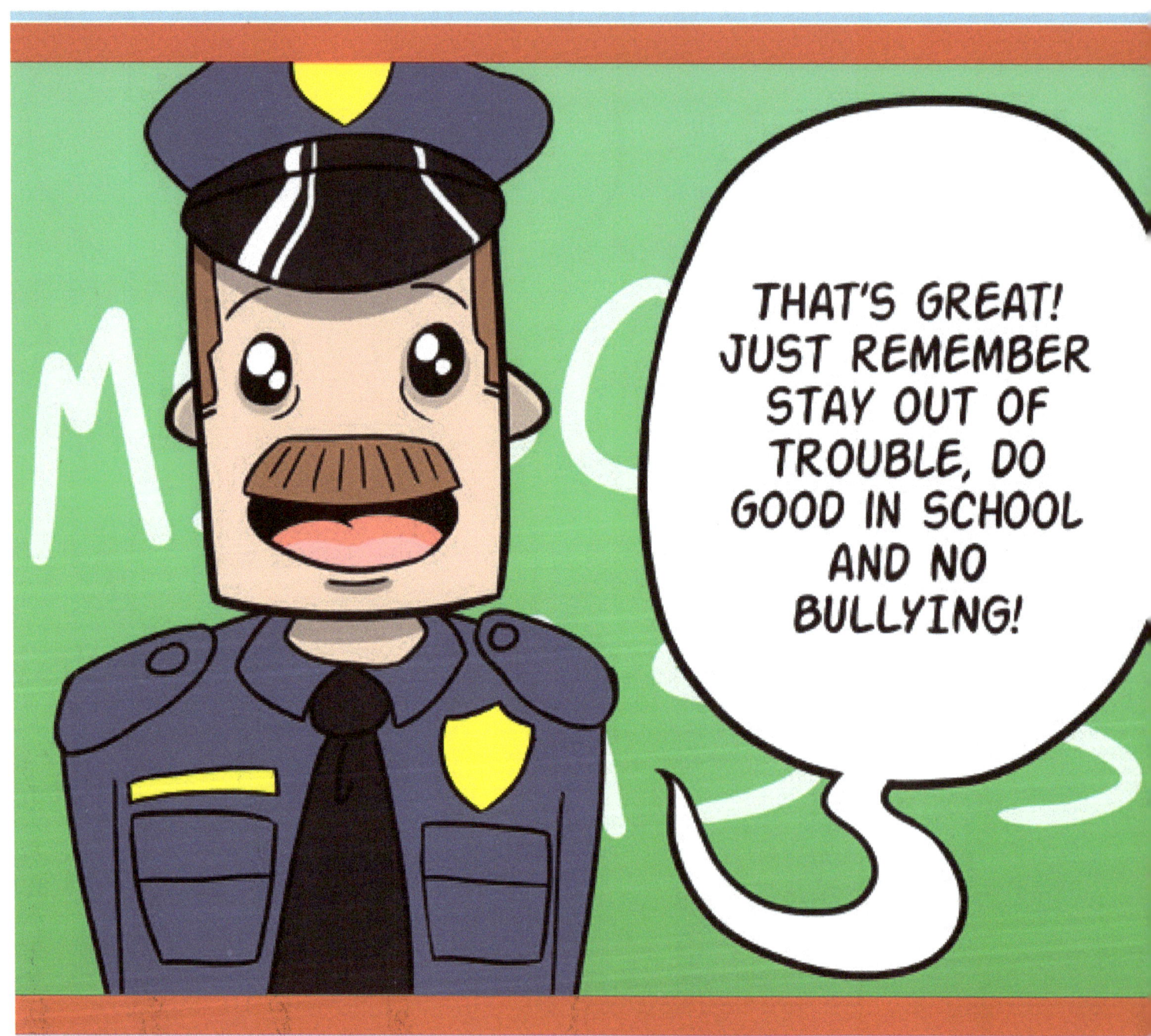

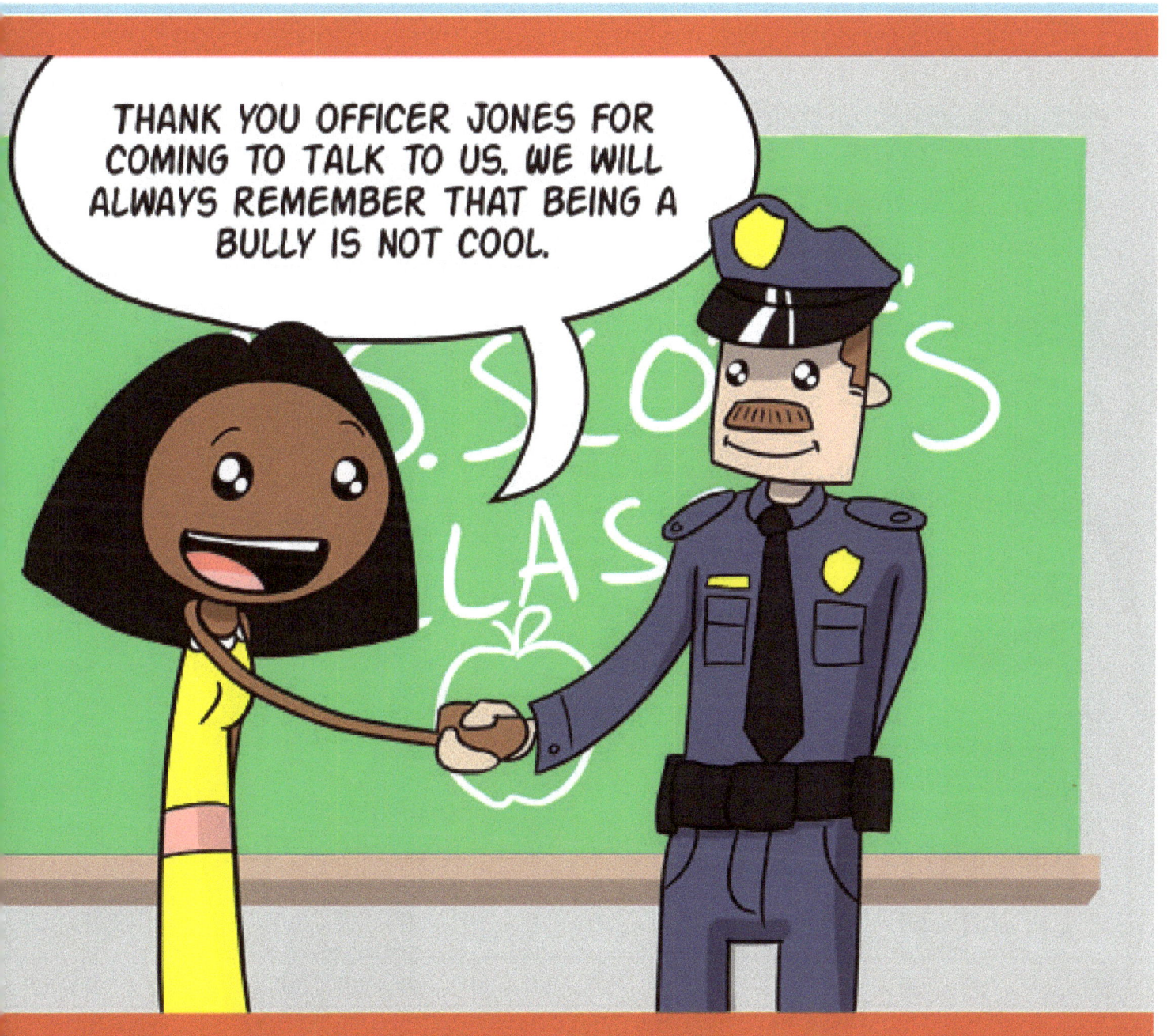

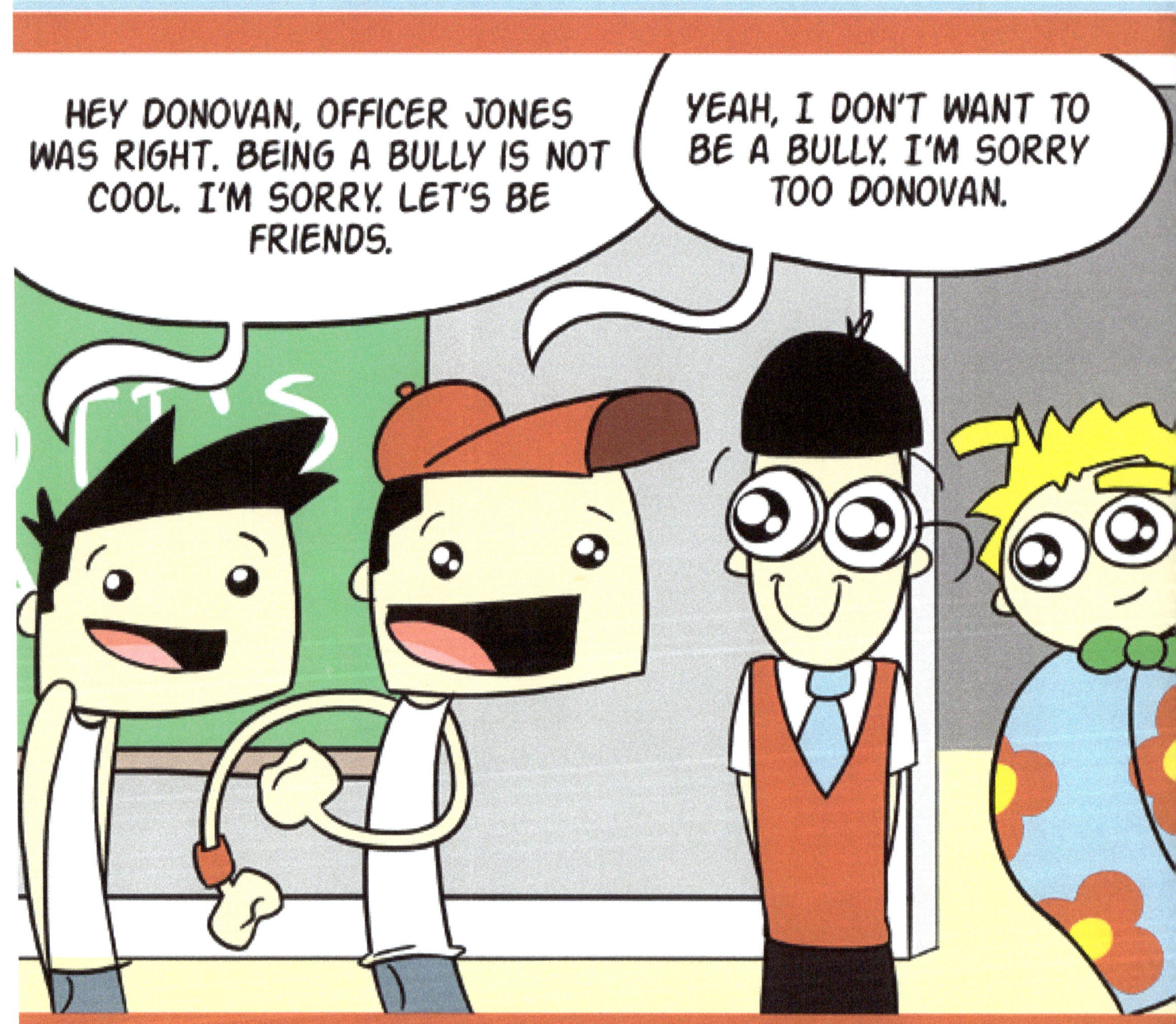

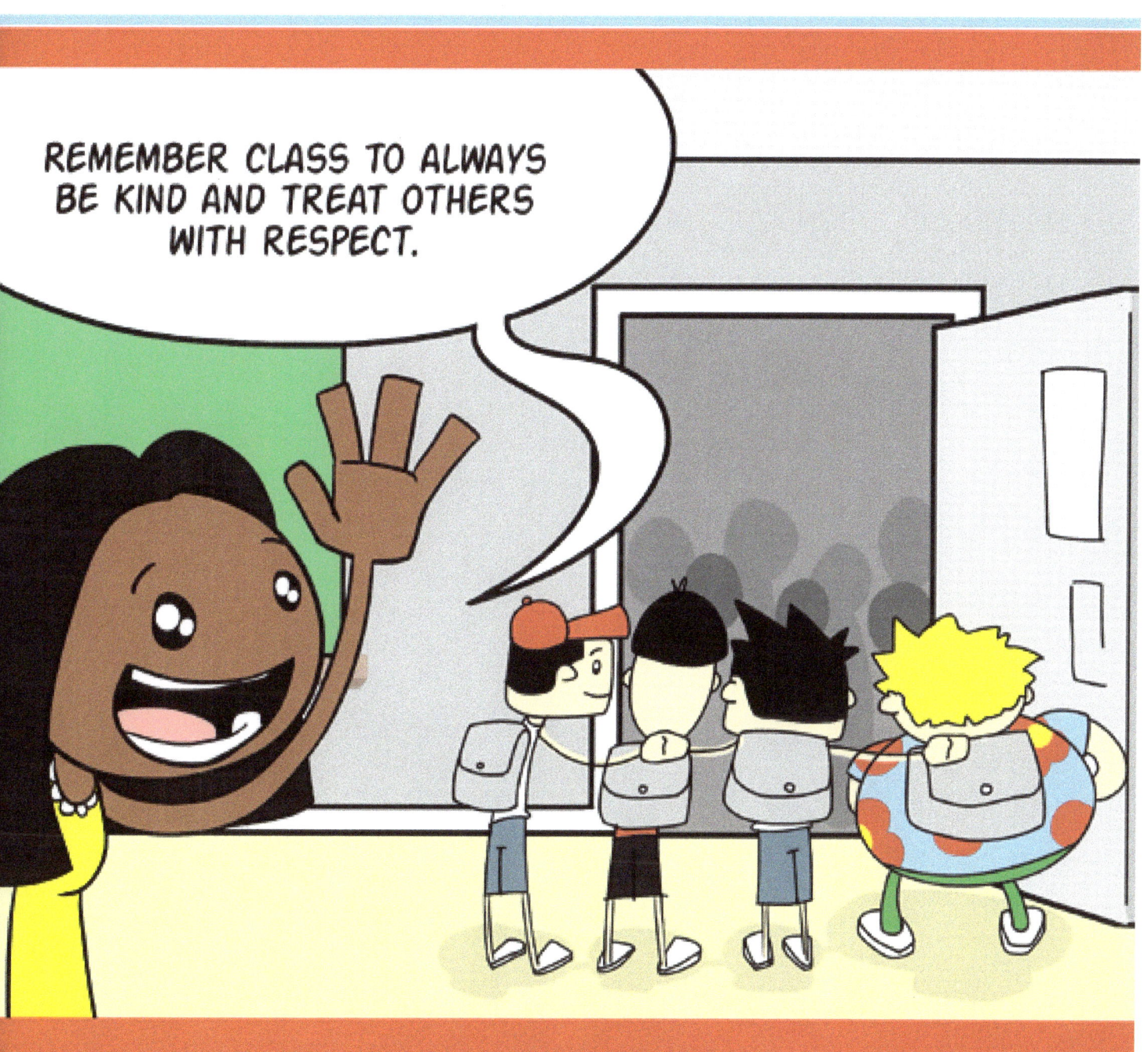